SLOW
JOGGING

SLOW JOGGING

Lose Weight, Stay Healthy, and Have Fun with Science-Based, Natural Running

HIROAKI TANAKA, PhD
and MAGDALENA JACKOWSKA

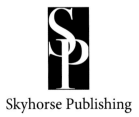

Skyhorse Publishing

Skyhorse Publishing books may be purchased in bulk at special discounts for sales promotion, corporate gifts, fund-raising, or educational purposes. Special editions can also be created to specifications. For details, contact the Special Sales Department, Skyhorse Publishing, 307 West 36th Street, 11th Floor, New York, NY 10018 or info@skyhorsepublishing.com.

Skyhorse® and Skyhorse Publishing® are registered trademarks of Skyhorse Publishing, Inc.®, a Delaware corporation.

Visit our website at www.skyhorsepublishing.com.

10 9 8 7 6 5 4 3

Library of Congress Cataloging-in-Publication Data is available on file.

Cover design by Tom Lau
Cover photo credit: iStockphoto
Photo credits introduction: Mark Cucuzzella

Print ISBN: 978-1-5107-5362-4
Ebook ISBN: 978-1-5107-0832-7

Printed in China

Table of Contents

Foreword: Jog Slow to Keep Running Healthy (and Fast too!)... vii

Chapter 1: Introduction 1

Chapter 2: Why Slow Jogging? 13

Chapter 3: Slow Jogging Basics 23

Chapter 4: All About *Niko Niko* Pace 37

Chapter 5: How Slow Jogging Improves Your Health and Well-being 45

Chapter 6: Weight Loss with Slow Jogging 59

Chapter 7: Self-Care and Injury Prevention 73

Chapter 8: Slow Jogging and Your First Marathon 83

Chapter 9: Slow Jogging for Experienced Runners 97

Chapter 10: Slow Jogging Success Stories 111

Chapter 11: Slow Jogging FAQs 123

Chapter 12: Final Thoughts for a Lifetime of Successful Slow Jogging 139

Slow Jogging: References 143

For More Information About the Slow Jogging Movement 151

Acknowledgments 153

Jog Slow to Keep Running Healthy (and Fast too!)

One of the most inspiring scientists and self-experimenting athletes alive today is my good friend, Japanese running guru Dr. Hiro Tanaka. Dr. Tanaka has changed my life and his message now is being shared with the U.S. Air Force to help create injury-free and more fit Airmen. I had the privilege of first meeting Dr. Tanaka, a Professor at Fukuoka University in Japan, at the Boston Marathon in 2011 after I gave a talk on minimal running and the benefits of running "easy." Dr. Tanaka showed me his heart rate and pace progression from building endurance, learning good form, and reducing his dependence on a running shoe. It led to his clocking in a 2:38 marathon at age fifty plus. This comes after reversing dyslipidemia, which was his inspiration to start running again. Dr. Tanaka later came as a guest to the US in 2012 for one of my Healthy Running courses and gave a community talk on "slow jogging." In front of everyone, he demonstrated this easy and relaxed movement which almost anyone can do safely.

He also gave me a copy of his book, originally published in Japanese, and whose title translated in English means "Run with Smile, Midfoot Strike." Like Dr. Tanaka, I am a big believer in "slow jogging" as a foundation for fitness and health. Any runner can master this technique to develop a soft and springy landing. You have to deserve to run hard and fast. Use "slow jogging" for recovery too; barefoot is best for this, in my opinion, to fully recover.

Dr. Tanaka's approach is a throwback to what Bill Bowerman wrote about in his 1967 bestselling book *Jogging*, which came out nearly a half-century ago. Bowerman talked about easy running as the best way to train the cardiac, respiratory, and circulatory systems. Bowerman also mentioned that for beginners, a walk/run style was ideal to start with. For those who are new to the fitness routine, running is likely to be intense; however, as people become more fit walking is not strenuous enough. So learning the skill of jogging will pay dividends as you become fitter, and eventually can spend more time jogging and less walking.

Here is how Bowerman defined jogging:

1. Jogging means a steady or an easy-paced running, while alternating with breath catching between periods of walking.
2. It means a kind of running, generally a slow regular trot that has been described as the next step up from walking.
3. Jogging describes the entire program of physical fitness outlined in this book.

Bowerman's *Jogging*—used copies of the out-of-print book can be found online at Amazon.com and elsewhere—went on to set the sample and safe plan which was used for cardiac patients by legendary coach Arthur Lydiard in New Zealand. The tables and charts are timeless and will progress almost anyone to thirty minutes of slow jogging in twelve weeks.

With *Slow Jogging*, Dr. Tanaka is expanding on the same foundation that Bowerman established, and millions of American followed. *Jogging* was a best-seller and sold over one million copies. Perhaps that same kind of success awaits Dr. Tanaka. For the time being anyway, the message for many runners is to simply "slow down!"

Here is my slow jogging journey. At forty-nine years old, it is never too late to learn new things and share with others. Although slowing now with age and new priorities, my average completion time of twenty Boston finishes is 2:36. Along the way, I have also compiled twenty-two Marine Corps finishes with an average of 2:38.

Looking back at these marathons has given me a new perspective on running. In today's culture there is a trend and emphasis on high-intensity training as the path to success. I agree that for immediate performance this is true, but the jury is out if we are talking about long-term health and balance if one has a busy life. There are also lots of folks who read stuff, write stuff, and make claims as to what is true based on short term results, but have never actually run.

The late Dr. George Sheehan wrote "we are all an experiment of one." This is true, but I think one must understand the principles of overall health and how to treat your body to keep the experiment going. Since my foot surgeries in 2000, I have not done any training which would be considered "hard" or "anaerobic" by modern extreme fitness zealots. Most proponents of "pain is gain" cannot produce this type of sustainable performance data in themselves or any of their clients or athletes. I have not missed a Boston or Marine Corps since 2000 (and have not had running-related injury since then either) and despite some years of extreme weather at these races, the times are all consistent with the gentle physiologic age-related decline.

Below is a photo of my first marathon, the Marine Corps Marathon in 1988. I was in my first year of medical school and had taken the summer off of running after four years of competitive running in college and the toll it took on my body. I also lived in LA that summer and tried to run one day but found the air so bad my lungs actually hurt.

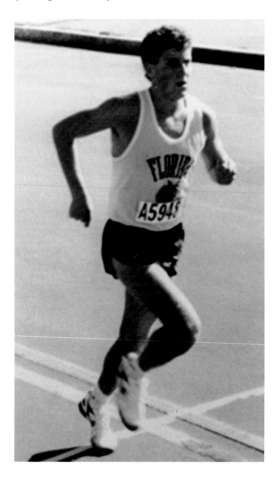

I quickly put on twenty pounds as I did not change my diet from the typical "runner's diet" of low fat and high carbs (notice a bit bulkier body). On return to medical school, I again found the joy in jogging for stress relief and to allow me to concentrate better in studies. One day I joined a friend for a long run and ended up running about sixteen miles. He convinced me to line up with him in D.C. two weeks later where I finished in 2:34 in my minimal Nike Duelists. I was hooked.

Unfortunately, I wore these same shoes in Boston the following spring to fly down the hills in the first half of the race (a 1:08 split), but my quads were mashed potatoes by Boston College. So I wound up taking the T home for one of my only two marathon DNFs. Learned that lesson! (My other DNF was in NYC in 1991 when I lined up with severe plantar fasciitis). I wore an old Florida Track Club singlet given to me by my Loyola High School coach Phil Kirby since I did not feel like I had returned to fitness as a runner worthy of representing my university or the U.S.\ Air Force.

This next finish photo is two years later, in 1990, when I was chasing my first sub 2:30. In those years, the Marine Corps Race finished on top of Iwo Jima and my sub 2:30 evaporated with the Hains Point winds (miles 20–23 used to be there). Add to that the steep last half-mile climb, and I finished in 2:31. I once again felt like a runner and wore my college colors (University of Virginia), and even the painter's cap with the bill flipped up in homage to Dick Beardsley who ran Alberto Salazar to the line at Boston a few years prior.

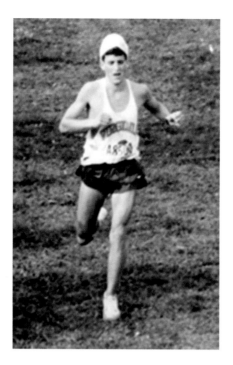

Here is me running happily at the 2014 Air Force Marathon. Note my Garmin watch—in other words, a smile on my wrist, another principle of Dr. Tanaka's "Run with Smile." I won this race in both 2006 and 2011, and have a string of thirteen top 10 finishes here. I have finished well over a hundred marathons all under three hours (except the two DNFs) and multiple ultras and have not worn my knees out, the eternal curse of so many runners.

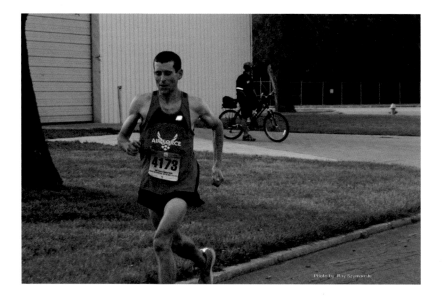

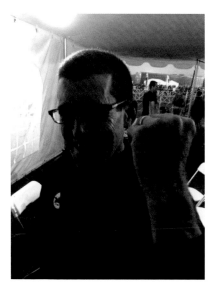

So what is the "secret sauce" of long-term healthy running?

- Slow down!
- Run for joy
- Recover
- Do not run too hard
- Finish each run as if you could do it again
- Keep fast and agile with short sprints and drills
- Keep mobile, especially in the ankles and hips
- Keep your foundation strong—this is your foot. Wear flat shoes shaped like your foot to stand, walk, run, and play.
- Go barefoot as often as you can.
- Learn the skill of running and keep trying to master this. A tool like TrueForm motor-less treadmill helps.
- Do simple strength training with Kettle Bells and Burpees
- Be your own body sensor and coach
- Don't sit
- Eat real food
- Do not put pain into your body
- And pass it forward—we all continue to learn by teaching and sharing with others.

As of early 2016, we are training the U.S. Air Force Basic Trainees to "slow jog" for their "self-paced runs." These runs used to be efforts where the Airman felt compelled to stay with the lead group or pick a group running faster than they should based on the culture of military fitness where you must push every day. The results of this mode of training is off-the-chart musculoskeletal injuries. So we are reversing this now and teaching the principle of "master the art of slow jogging" before loading it up with speed and power.

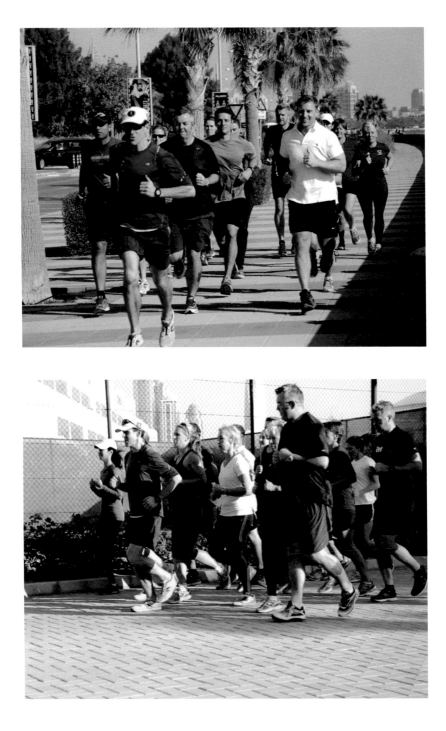

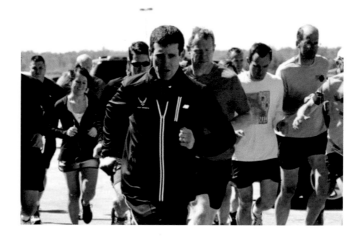

By training in this manner, I just performed a VO2 max test at age forty-nine of 65 mil/kg/min, the highest score for any age at the military facility where I just tested. For frame of reference, as of January 2016, this facility has performed over 1,000 tests. People ask me how I train and I tell them "slow and relaxed," spicing it up with a few short sprints (but never to the point of fatigue). I thank Dr. Tanaka for giving me the courage to continue to train this way.

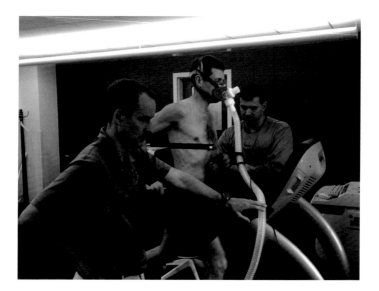

It is everyone's birthright to run. There is something magical about both feet being in the air at the same time. In my community, through our running store, Two Rivers Treads, we teach this method at every Couch to 5K or new runner workshop. Smiles go around the room as participants try this, release their tension, and forgo the impression that running needs to be painful.

Ready to feel this yourself? Then you've selected the right book: *Slow Jogging* will change your life and, through sharing, the life of others who wish to live the vigorous life through the ages.

—Mark Cucuzzella, MD

Professor, West Virginia University School of Medicine, Lieutenant Colonel, U.S. Air Force, and Race Director, Freedom's Run

CHAPTER 1

Introduction

Running is America's most popular participatory sport. The number of races and runners is at the highest in history, and the trend is unlikely to change anytime soon.

At the same time, large numbers of runners get injured—nearly half in any given year, according to some estimates. What should be an enjoyable activity is often one filled with pain, or becomes an abandoned pursuit. Most runners get injured because they are going too fast too soon, are overtraining, have faulty running form, and/or are wearing improper footwear.

Other people want to become runners, but never even get to the point where they do enough to get injured. They've been told "no pain, no gain," and think that exercise should be hard work all the time. To them, running feels like an unenjoyable chore. Despite their best intentions, they're unable to stick with it.

There has to be a better, more efficient, healthier, and pain-free approach to running—especially one that will appeal to beginners and runners of all shapes and ages.

Distinguished exercise researcher and veteran runner Hiroaki Tanaka, PhD, who is known as Japan's running guru and is the author of several sports science books, has found that way. His licensed method, known as "slow jogging," is ideal for injury-free running. It also helps participants lose weight faster and prevent and treat many lifestyle diseases, such as type 2 diabetes. Slow jogging is a healthier and natural way to run.

Slow Jogging is a timely and useful update to legendary track coach and Nike co-founder Bill Bowerman's bestselling book *Jogging,* which was published nearly a half-century ago and has sold more than one million copies. That book launched America's first running boom. We hope that *Slow Jogging* will convince many more Americans to take up running—whether for health and fitness reasons, to lose weight, to limit wear and tear on the body, or just to have fun. This book will tell you all you need to know to improve your life through an effective but sustainable workout program.

In Japan, you will see people slow jogging everywhere, and you'll see all kinds of people doing it. You'll see the elderly, moving at two-to-three miles per hour, which for many people is close to walking speed. There are also busy businessmen, who know that five minutes of jogging a few times a day can be as beneficial to their health as twenty or thirty minutes of continuous exercise. Then there are experienced runners who alternate intense training with slow jogging, giving their bodies a chance to recover and reminding themselves of the pure, childish joy of running in fresh air, which tends to get lost in serious training schedules. There is even Japanese Empress Michiko, who appeared on national TV on the day of her eighty-first birthday and explained that she jogs every day to stay in good health.

The key to slow jogging is what we call *niko niko* pace. In Japanese, *niko niko* means "smile." Unlike traditional training, which requires concentration and effort, slow jogging is more like taking a walk, at an intensity light enough to enjoy conversation or, if you're by yourself, to just smile. Slow jogging also gives you a rare opportunity to spend time with friends and family, or to refocus in solitude. While having such a good time, you will not notice the time passing and calories burned.

In this book, we'll show you how to use this powerful method to achieve your fitness goals, whether they have to do with weight loss, improving health, getting faster, having fun, or, the best of all options, all of the above.

Before we dive in to the many ways that slow jogging can improve your life, here's a little background on the authors of this book, Hiroaki Tanaka and Magdalena Jackowska. We hope that by our sharing how we came to embrace slow jogging, you'll view us not as elites preaching to you, but fellow runners you can trust as your guides.

Hiroaki Tanaka, PhD

My life as a runner started in my elementary school days. Tokyo was chosen to host the 1964 Olympics, and children across the nation took interest in sports, dreaming of participating in the event. I felt enthusiastic about running and took my first steps on the track. Over the years, I started training more seriously, and in high school I specialized in distances between 400 and 1500 meters. Back then, however, I had many injuries and no spectacular results.

Like most young runners in Japan, I dreamed of participating in the Hakone Ekiden, one of the most prominent relay marathons for university students, not to mention one of the most famous sporting events in Japan. It was the main reason why I eventually turned to long-distance running after entering the university.

I put my heart and soul into training, only to soon find out that my body wasn't quite able to keep up. The cycle of injuries, the recovery, and the frantic training continued until I ended up in the university hospital for a complete body health check. I was diagnosed with an innate heart condition that disqualified me from further training. I was allowed to do only low-intensity light exercise, such as walking and easy gymnastics. I was only nineteen years old.

Brokenhearted, I couldn't get track and field out of my mind, and became a team manager for the students running in the Hakone Ekiden. After graduation I decided to continue my studies at the university to research the field of physiology of exercise and endurance training, such as easy exercise prescriptions to improve cardiovascular functions.

As the years passed, I researched the field of sports science but didn't really have a lot of time to run or exercise myself. In the meantime, I became quite nervous about my health, and whenever I felt tired, I associated it with my heart disease.

At the age of thirty-seven, I lived in Montreal for my sabbatical year. I was there doing a collaborative study on the harmful influence of hard exercise such as all-out marathons. We didn't have enough subjects in our experiment, so I wanted to participate as both researcher and subject. I didn't have all those small tasks that kept me so busy back in Japan, so I resumed running. I jogged slowly for an hour every day, usually covering five to six miles.

The 1984 Montreal Marathon was my first time to experience running with thousands of other runners, and it felt incredible. I was doing really well in the first half, probably faster than eight minutes per mile, but from then on my legs felt heavier and heavier and I wasn't able to keep my speed. Other runners, even some much older than me, started passing me. From the 21-mile marker, I was literally dragging my heavy legs and eventually walked my way to the finish line. My finishing time was 4:11. I was pretty sure that was the first and last marathon of my life.

After returning to Japan, I was again too busy for more than a slow weekend jog of two and a half to three miles every now and then. I led a mostly sedentary life and started putting on weight.

On my forty-fifth birthday the scale showed twenty-two more pounds than in my school days. A health check showed that I was also suffering also from fatty liver and high cholesterol. I felt like a doctor neglecting his own health.

After that wake-up call, things started to turn around. I was asked to become an advisor of a semi-professional Ekiden team and a group of runners preparing for the 1993 Honolulu Marathon. I knew it was my chance to take on the marathon once again, and see how my theories would work in practice. I decided to run a marathon for the second time.

My training consisted mostly of a three-mile jog once or twice a week. I tried to predict my results scientifically with an incremental test: Running at gradually increased speed and verifying my body's reaction. To my huge surprise, having barely been running a total monthly distance of twenty miles, I came up with a highly unbelievable estimated time of 3:30 to 3:45.

In the race, considering that I hardly ever ran longer distances, around Mile 6 I got seriously anxious. I kept running, repeating to myself a mantra: "Believe in science. Don't give up." Dr. Peter A. Farrell, a specialist in the field of running performance, had proved that scientific estimations of marathon finishing time were quite accurate. I wound up finishing in 3:30:03. Unlike in my first marathon, the second time I managed to run at a constant pace. In the second half I felt slightly tired, but not to the extent that would force me to slow. I felt quite comfortable and confident overall.

Nine years had passed since my first marathon at the age of thirty-seven, so getting slower would have been perfectly natural. I also was more than twenty pounds heavier than nine years earlier. Despite all that, my time was more than forty minutes better. I did some calculations right away. Going back to my weight from my university days, I could become light enough and therefore fast enough to break 3:00 in my next marathon.

The following year, after weight reduction and training based on slow jogging, I did so. In my sixth marathon, in Aoshima, Japan, I finished in 2:55:11.

That was when I started thinking about running technique. I was inspired by the way sprinters effectively use the springs in their feet by landing on the midfoot/forefoot, and I applied their technique to distance running. My usual runs at a slow pace allowed me to work on modifying my technique, and year by year I steadily improved my results. In 1998, at the age of fifty, my big dream came true and I completed a marathon under 2:40. That result qualified me for the elite Betsudai Marathon in Oita, Japan. There, in my eighteenth marathon, I ran my personal best of 2:38:50.

More than thirty years have passed since I ran my first marathon, which at the time I thought would be my last. Since then I have completed sixty-five marathons in thirteen countries, some fun and some as serious races. My running technique—the one we'll describe in detail later in this book—has kept me injury-free. My next dream is to run a sub-3:00 marathon at the age of seventy.

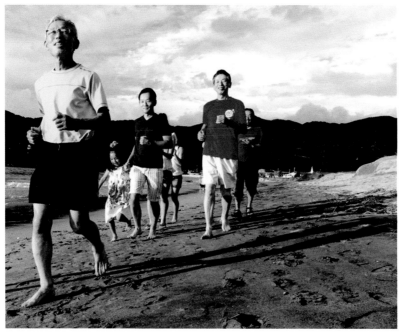

Credit: Chie Nakamura

A footnote: At the age of twenty-five, I had my heart re-examined. It turned out that what had been diagnosed as a heart condition was really the result of my poor diet and too-strenuous exercise. So there never was a reason for me to stop competitive running in the first place. With today's ultrasonography techniques, a similar mistake would never happen now, but back then the wrong diagnosis became the reason I gave up my career in sport and focused on research instead. Many years later, that led to creating the *niko niko* pace and slow jogging theories you'll learn in this book.

Magdalena Jackowska

Unlike Professor Tanaka, sport hasn't always been an important part of my life. Quite the contrary, actually. At school I was at least one head shorter than everybody else in the class and was always the last one to be picked for a team in Physical Education. I went to school one year earlier, so being smaller and weaker was only natural, but for many years it became both a reason and an excuse to dislike sport in general. As an adolescent I started to enjoy occasional solo exercise, usually cycling or hiking, but my lack of interest in team sports never changed. And I held the typical opinion of sport in general. Training, competition, pushing myself harder than felt good, sweat and tears—that was my image of sport, and I didn't like it.

Things started to change after I moved to Japan. I was twenty-four and living in Fukuoka, near Ohori Park, which, as I would later find out, was a mecca to the local runners. I would see them every day of the year, through the sweaty, humid summer and freezing, windy winter, at every hour of day and night. Intrigued, one evening I tried jogging on the 1.2-mile path around the pond in the park. Pretty soon, going there for a lap or two every other week became my new routine. As with most enthusiastic beginners, I never thought about my technique. That happened only after a chance encounter with Professor Tanaka.

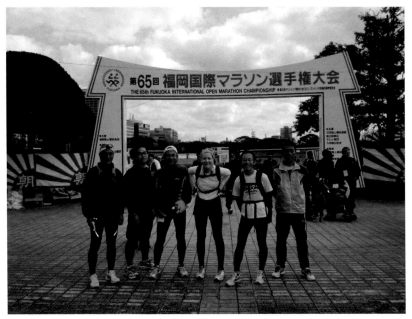

Credit: Magdalena Jackowska

Thanks to him, I gradually came to love slow jogging, which represented everything I enjoy about exercise, without the pressure, competition, and hard-core training that made me avoid sport for many years. Luckily for me, it happened early enough in my running life to prevent me from most of the typical beginner's mistakes and also kept me free from suffering from injuries and burnout.

Now, more than five years later, I can honestly say that meeting Professor Tanaka and discovering slow jogging changed my life. In the meantime, I started to work at the Institute for Physical Activity, at Fukuoka University, helping Professor Tanaka with his research and learning more about health and fitness. Before I knew it, slow jogging—its theory and practice—became my passion and lifestyle.

In 2013, we introduced slow jogging to my home country, Poland. The following year, the first Polish book on slow jogging was published. The ever-growing number of slow jogging fans and media attention in Poland was incredible.

Together with all the work-related activities as slow jogging instructor and promoter, I continue to enjoy slow jogging myself. Unlike Professor Tanaka, I will probably always be far from becoming a fast, goal-oriented runner, nor do I have a marathon runner's physique. But I still enjoy races and in my relatively short running career I have run more than twenty marathons and ultramarathons on different continents—for the fun, for the experience, for the adventure. My best marathon time of 3:40:40 is more a side result from my commitment to the slow jogging lifestyle than my main goal.

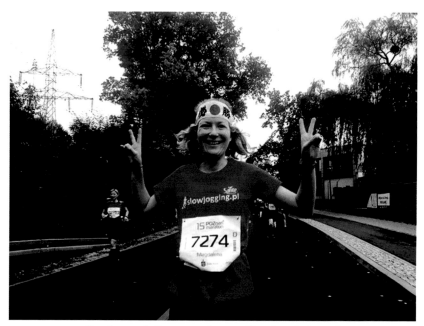

Magda completing a marathon, smiling the whole way!

My jogging story might not be spectacular, but even without extreme weight loss and impressive personal records, slow jogging is one of the best things that ever happened to me, as it has been to hundreds of other people I've met along the way. If you give it a try, I'm pretty sure you will be able to say the same, and sooner than you think.

Toward that end, let's look in detail at what exactly slow jogging is. That's the focus of the next chapter.

CHAPTER 2
Why Slow Jogging?

What is the world's most basic, accessible, and ubiquitous form of physical activity that doesn't require equipment or company?

We can all agree that this is walking and running. No doubt these are great ways to stay fit and healthy, and easy to incorporate into our everyday lives. Unfortunately, they are not universally effective and cannot be universally recommended.

First, let's agree that any physical activity is better than no activity at all. However, if you do decide to exercise, why not investigate your options and choose wisely?

Despite all of the benefits of running, it can be exhausting, and is often the best choice only for those who are young and already fairly fit. And let's be honest—many adults simply hate running.

Walking, on the other hand, is pleasant, but for most people is done at too low an intensity to be considered exercise; that can lead to health improvements or weight loss.

What would be the perfect middle ground? An activity that is equally accessible, not too strenuous but intense enough to be effective? Light enough for you to enjoy it and not give up but still powerful when working on your dream body and fitness goals?

You probably guessed by now—jogging. More precisely, slow jogging. Let's look at why that's the case.

We Are Born to Run

Humans are the best distance runners in the animal world. That was the breakthrough thesis presented in *Nature* in 2004 by anthropologists Dennis Bramble and Daniel Lieberman, who theorized that evolution designed us to run.

Up until about ten thousand years ago, humans mainly got their food by hunting with their bare hands. There are still tribes in Africa living as hunters and gatherers. Research shows that, every day, they first walk for close to twenty miles until they find their prey, and then chase it for three to five hours at a speed of around six miles per hour. Just like other animals, historically, humans chose to run when they needed to move fast. Even during the New Stone Age, when humanity settled and began to live a more stationary life based on agriculture and stock-farming, there was still a need to hurry and run on an everyday basis.

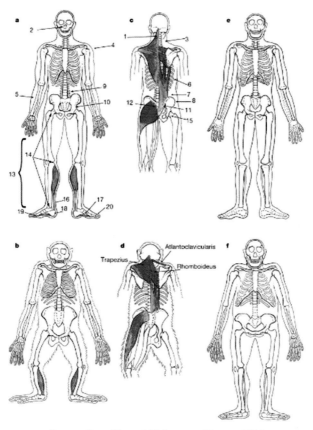

Source: Bramble and Lieberman, Nature, 2004

Even our basic human anatomy makes it clear that our bodies are designed to run rather than walk. If we compare ourselves to chimpanzees—the species most closely related to us—our legs are longer, while the pelvis is shorter and wider. Further, the Achilles tendon is longer, and the back and gluteus muscles are better developed. We have arched feet, which are absent in chimpanzees. During running, the elastic structures of the feet exert propulsive force and absorb the shock of the landing.

All these features make running the most natural movement for humans. Thanks to the shorter pelvis, for example, the abdominal part of our bodies (the region between the thorax and ilium) allows us to twist our upper bodies and our legs to widen like compasses. These actions are crucial in making our strides longer and thus increasing speed when running, but aren't necessary in regular walking. The Achilles tendon is barely used while walking, but during running it helps legs work like springs and improves the effectiveness of locomotion. Similarly, gluteus muscles are not necessary to walk, but are essential for running.

There are other adaptations that allow humans to continue to run in conditions that eventually make other animals stop. Our ability to sweat, as well as our hairlessness, and our ability to breathe through our mouths, all are essential traits that allow us to get rid of excess heat whilst pursuing game in the hottest part of the day.

All those physiological features and more have made us fantastic endurance athletes. Many animals beat us in sprints, but we have always been the world's best distance runners.

Out of Touch With Our Heritage

Nowadays, some of us still cover impressive distances daily, although usually it's to get ready for a marathon, rather than out of necessity. But for the most part, the majority of people in developed countries don't get enough exercise from their day-to-day lives.

Contrast that with the situation in Kenya, which produces more than half of the world's best marathoners. In the Rift Valley area, where most of the great Kenyan runners grow up, elementary school children can cover several miles per day. This is all done in a combination of walking and jogging while going to and from school. Chores such as fetching water and tending to livestock can mean more distance covered.

The situation for Japanese school children used to be similar. For example, at one of the oldest elementary schools in Fukuoka, the longest distance from home to school was almost four miles from the school's creation in 1873 up until 1970. But in the following decade, the distance shrunk to one mile. Since then, children in the area have lost the habit of physical activity as something that's a natural part of their day.

Similarly, in the United States, 70 percent of the population was still working long, hard hours to produce food at the turn of the twentieth century. Children of this era walked several miles to school, while now they are taken by car or bus as close as possible to the school entrance.

How Slow Jogging Relates to Our Running Heritage

When done correctly, slow jogging is similar to how our ancestors used to cover several miles without getting tired. How is that possible? The answer lies in physiology, especially of muscles.

Our muscles are composed of thin fibers of two different types, referred to as slow-twitch and fast-twitch. Fast-twitch muscle fibers are crucial in intense sports such as sprint, jumps, and throws, while slow-twitch fibers are what are mostly used in endurance pursuits such as long-distance running, Nordic skiing, and cycling.

Fast-twitch muscle fibers produce energy instantly, but cause rapid drop in glucose levels, leading to lactate accumulation and increased fatigue. Lactate is a byproduct of metabolizing glucose for energy; its presence is linked to lowered available energy sources and leads to exhaustion. Contraction of slow-twitch fibers takes longer, but they are more durable and accumulate lactate more slowly.

During physical exercise the number of muscle fibers increases with speed. Therefore, during very slow jogging the energy comes mainly from contractions of slow-twitch fibers and their number increases to maximum at *niko niko* pace. At a faster pace, fast-twitch muscles are activated and their number also increases with speed.

Slow jogging at *niko niko* pace activates the greatest number of slow-twitch fibers, without activating the fast-twitch ones. That's why it's possible to continue exercising for a long time with no fatigue or running out of breath. We are slightly simplifying the process here, but thanks to regular, slow exercise, slow-twitch fibers work more effectively and part of them changes their nature, which results in lower lactate accumulation even for faster running.

Jogging vs. Walking

There are situations when we break into a run, and quite often they have nothing to with the willingness to exercise. Think about traffic lights changing to red or being late to an extremely important meeting. We all instinctively choose running over walking when moving at a higher speed.

There are some speeds at which it's possible to either walk or run. So when do we actually start to run? Interestingly, when increasing the speed on the treadmill, the moment when we switch from walking to running is quite similar for all of us. According to research by Alan Hreljac, published in 1993 in *Medicine and Science in Sports and Exercise*, it's 4.6±0.28 miles per hour in America, and about four miles per hour in Japan.

Walking at a speed up to just before three miles per hour is extremely efficient, but at 3.7 miles per hour and faster it gets exponentially worse. You would think that switching from walking to running at a given speed (referred to as preferred transition speed) happens unconsciously for reasons of better efficiency. It turns out that, although walking is still more efficient, we switch to running.

Hreljac also investigated how tired we feel when walking and running at different intensities by using the famous rating of perceived exertion (RPE) scale developed by Gunnar Borg from Sweden. Despite requiring higher energy expenditure, running was thought to be equally tiring as walking and expressed with a similar number on the RPE scale.

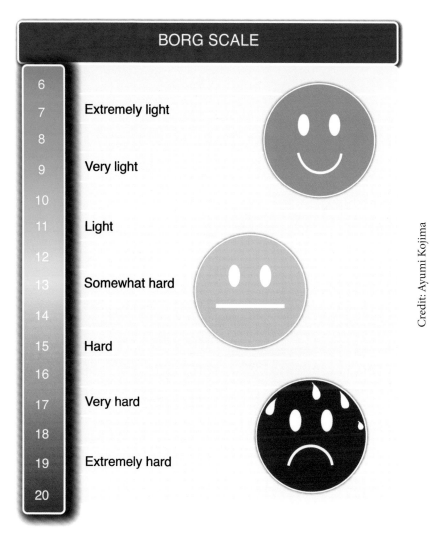

Credit: Ayumi Kojima

When moving slowly, we unconsciously choose walking as the more efficient mode of locomotion. However, if we intentionally switch to running (more specifically, very slow jogging), we are going to need more energy (and burn more calories) but will feel no more tired than when walking. To put it simply: when walking or jogging at the same, low speed, you'll burn many more calories in the same amount of time if you jog.

What's more, because running speed and energy expenditure are in linear relation, the physiological efficiency of running is the same at every speed, from slow jogging to sprinting. The calories that you burn with every mile are exactly the same, whether it takes you thirty minutes or six minutes to cover a mile.

Slow Jogging Is Enjoyable and Doable

When asked "Do you like running?," the vast majority of adults will answer with a resounding "no." The answer would likely be the same if it was asked about jogging. The essential reason: Most people would say, "running is hard." Even among regular runners, many don't find it enjoyable. They think it's difficult, and they think that's the way it's supposed to be.

So not only running but even jogging, which used to be an essential activity in human lives, is now generally disliked for being "hard."

As noted above, when moving faster and faster, humans will likely start running at around 7 METs on the intensity scale, which means seven times the intensity of rest. Even though that's the speed when we start running instinctively, for many of us it already constitutes hard exercise, outside of our comfort zone. According to a recent National Health and Nutrition Examination Survey, running will be labeled as "hard" for as many as 20 to 40 percent of American men and 60 to 70 percent of American women between twenty and forty-nine years old.

Remember, our ancestors chased the prey for three to five hours at six miles per hour. For them, a jog at three to four miles per hour would have been a piece of cake.

We, however, living in the twenty-first century, have extremely comfortable lives that make physical activity almost unnecessary. As a result, we have possibly the lowest average fitness level in human history; no wonder jogging is "hard."

But contrary to popular belief, you don't have to work through the pain. Slow down enough to feel at ease. And just keep going—with a smile! Soon you'll have increased your fitness and feel again like elementary school children, the vast majority of whom say they like running.

And another reason to slow down to a speed at which you're comfortable: to experience the so-called runner's high.

In the 1990s, studies showed that our bodies have the ability to produce a marijuana-like substance (endocannabinoids) that regulates a variety of physiological processes, including feeling pleasure and neutralizing pain. Researchers were wondering whether and what kind of physical activity can induce their production.

First, researchers were able to confirm that this high happens when running and climbing. A recent study, described further in Chapter 5, checked the concentration of endocannabinoids in blood after a session of walking, slow jogging, medium-pace jogging, and running, and found out that walking didn't lead to endocannabinoids production, slow jogging resulted in a remarkable number, and medium-pace jogging led to a slight increase; meanwhile, running didn't induce their production at all.

It might have been a physiological reward after a long, slow jog, such as after three to five hours of hunting for our ancestors. The same enjoyable endocannabinoid experience is available to you through regular slow jogging at your *niko niko* pace.

What exactly is slow jogging? How in practice is it different from regular jogging or running? We'll look at those questions in depth in the next chapter.

CHAPTER 3

Slow Jogging Basics

What do we mean by when we use the word "jogging?" Is it how fast or slow is the person going? Is he or she running? Is there a specific pace that defines jogging, as opposed to running? Is jogging simply another word for "slow running?" In this chapter we'll answer these important questions and look at other fundamentals of a healthy, sustainable approach to jogging.

The term "jogging" became widely used in the United States in the late 1960s, as it was a result of a popular book with the title *Jogging*. Its author was University of Oregon track coach and Nike cofounder Bill Bowerman. He had been exposed to jogging while on vacation in New Zealand with his college team. He took time off and went for some easy runs with legendary running coach Arthur Lydiard, who had trained several Olympic running champions. On weekends, Lydiard would invite locals to join him for "fitness and sociability" runs, or what he called jogging. Lydiard wanted New Zealanders to stop being sedentary and get some easy, non-strenuous exercise.

Bowerman enjoyed these easy runs, and lost ten pounds in the process. He was eager to spread the message about jogging to residents in Eugene, Oregon, where he lived and coached. When these jogging get-togethers became popular, Bowerman decided to broaden the message, and co-wrote the 126-page bestselling *Jogging* book with the help of a local cardiologist. One of their big concerns was that Americans were in fairly poor shape, as television and driving generally dominated their free time. (This sound familiar?)

Over a million copies of Bowerman's book were eventually sold. Jogging became a household word and activity. It's simple to see why. The book made jogging within reach for all Americans, whether they were fit or fat, young or old, husband or wife. The best way to explain this phenomenon is to read a passage from the book:

> Jogging is different from most popular physical fitness programs. Unlike weight lifting, isometric exercises, and calisthenics with their emphasis on muscle building, jogging works to improve the heart, lungs, and circulatory system. Other body muscles are exercised as well, but the great benefit comes from improving the way the heart and lungs work. After all, when you are past thirty, bulging biceps and pleasing pectorals may boost your ego, but your life and health depend upon how fit your heart and lungs are. Jogging is a simple type of exercise, requiring no highly developed skills. The great appeal is that it is so handy.

The book included three 12-week training plans, each one tailored to an individual's overall health, fitness level, and weight. Each plan combined jogging with some walking for the duration of the three-month period. The recommended average speed for joggers ranged from 15-minute miles to 7-minute miles.

There are other ways to define jogging than with a watch, as we will shortly demonstrate. Moreover, slow jogging means something much different than normal jogging. It's a bold rethinking of what it means to run healthy and injury-free. When you run too fast, you can damage your body, it can break down, and/or you can get injured or sick. If you're not running at all or doing only super light activity such as walking, that's not enough to markedly improve your health and fitness. The happy middle ground is slow jogging.

The word "jogging" itself implies that we are talking about a lower-intensity, slower movement than "running." However, most of us go for a "jog" and wind up exceeding our comfortable pace, making the whole experience tiring and discouraging. And that's a pity, because running at the right individually adjusted intensity is a wonderful way to stay fit and healthy. You'll lose weight, reduce stress, prevent illness, and improve brain function. And, believe it or not, within a year you will be able to run a marathon, if that's a goal you aspire to.

Let's examine some of the key concepts behind the slow jogging approach.

Number One Rule: Slow Down!

"I will begin running starting tomorrow!"

You may have said something like this at some point, and perhaps more than once. But then, if you're like most people, you made a crucial error—you ran at too high of an intensity and burned out quickly.

But why does this happen? It occurs simply because we have been long indoctrinated into the "no pain, no gain" approach to exercise. We expect to feel the burn. We want to feel the hurt. Because how else do we know we are working out? So we start too fast and begin to hate running just a few minutes into the experience. Getting out of breath, together with profuse sweating and a pounding heart, can discourage even the most determined beginners. How do you continue for thirty minutes or even begin to enjoy it?

There has to be a better way. First, you need to understand that no matter how low your fitness level is, it's very unlikely to be low enough to disqualify you from easy running. That is why you need to start slowly—really slowly. It's highly possible that, if you begin your running program at the proper intensity, you will be overtaken by walkers. Don't let this discourage you.

The key to success with slow jogging is to keep your individual *niko niko* pace. Remember, *niko niko* means "smile" in Japanese, and here is defined as an easy pace that you can keep with a smile. *Niko niko* pace varies greatly among both beginning and experienced runners. Later in the book we'll see how to find yours.

For complete beginners, it is recommended to start at an even lighter intensity, alternating one minute of slow jogging with thirty seconds of walking.

Landing Makes All the Difference

When walking, we usually land on our heel and push off with our forefoot in a basic heel-to-toe manner. When running, different patterns are possible—you can heel strike, as in walking, or you can forefoot strike. But which is better?

To answer that question, try this: Stand up and jump a couple of times, in a way that feels most natural. Now think about where you landed. Wasn't it the upper-central part of your foot? Now, try to jump and land on your heels. It might be painful and probably you will not be able to jump very high. When landing on your forefoot, the Achilles tendon gives you natural elasticity that helps you to spring off your feet and jump higher.

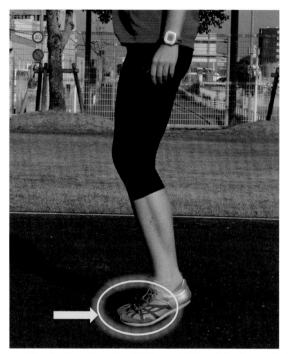

Jumping and forefoot landing. Credit: Kazumi Takeo, Magdalena Jackowska

Landing on your heels can cause a lot of pressure to your joints, especially the knees, and therefore increase the risk of some of the most common running injuries. That happens because the collision of the heel to the ground generates an initial impact force that is usually greater than in the case of a forefoot strike.

To feel and remember movement patterns, try jogging in place, jumping, jogging backwards or barefoot. That is when your feet move naturally, which is the movement you will aim at when jogging as well. Just be careful—do not try jogging on your tiptoes, but by using the upper-central, widest part of your foot.

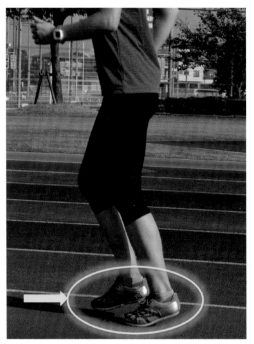

Credit: Kazumi Takeo, Magdalena Jackowska

Unfortunately, most of the modern running shoes, especially those designed for beginners, have a thick sole invented to minimize shocks resulting from landing on the heels. However, such a construction teaches you to land on the heel and inhibits the instinctive movement. Slow jogging and forefoot running require going back to basics and the instinctive way of running, so simple shoes with thin, elastic soles and a wide toe box, fitting well on the heel, are strongly recommended.

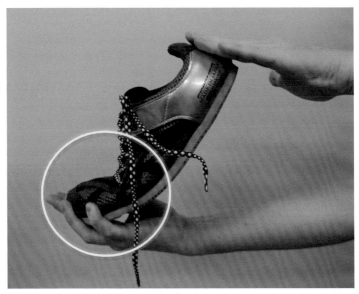

Simple shoes that are recommended for slow jogging. Credit: Kazumi Takeo,
Magdalena Jackowska

One more thing: If you are already a runner and you have always been a heel striker, midfoot might not always feel natural at first. Until it does, jog slowly to be able to focus on the way you land. A great way to learn is running barefoot or in barefoot-style shoes. Once you get used to midfoot striking, you should be able to do it in any kind of shoes.

Correct Posture

Now that you know how to land, it is time to move forward. Imagine that your body is a pole, straight from head to forefoot. Imagine that your legs are making small steps on two separate, parallel tracks. Make use of your Achilles tendon to take small jumps and land on the forefoot. Running or jogging is just a sequence of small jumps on alternate legs, so there is no need to kick or apply force to the ground. You will often see runners landing by putting their feet in a straight line; this is usually those trying to run faster by lengthening their strides.

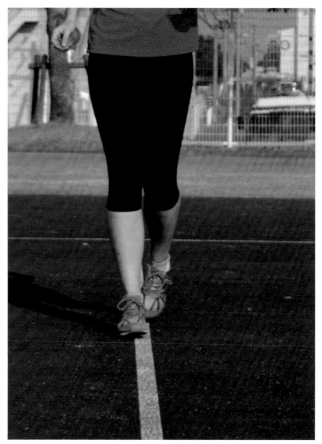

Incorrect running form. Credit: Kazumi Takeo

Doing so, however, means that these types of runners have to make extra body turns, which results in unnecessary energy loss. Further, turns of the pelvis are unavoidable in straight-line running and increase the stress on the knees and thus risk of injuries. Just like twisting a wire a number of times leads to it breaking, the extra turns with every single step can be quite harmful.

Think about babies: They begin to explore the world by crawling, later by standing up, and finally by walking and running, still with their legs slightly separated. Take a good look at how children naturally run and imitate their two-track movements.

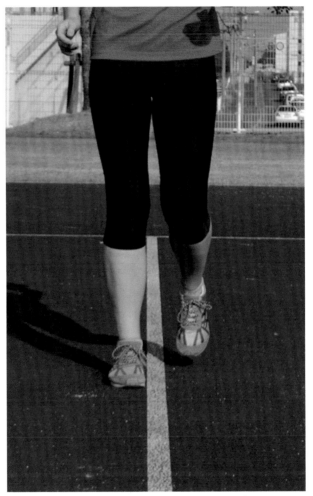

Correct running form. Credit: Kazumi Takeo

As far as the arms are concerned, you do not have to control them consciously. Form 90-degree angles with your elbows, clench your fists lightly imagining you are holding skiing poles, relax your shoulders, and swing your arms gently forward and back.

Pay attention to your whole body posture as well. Be careful not to draw in your chin; keep your head up in a neutral position. You should be straight in your hips and look at the road ahead of you, not your feet. Enjoying the view is part of the fun!

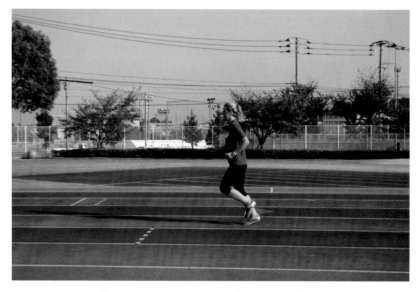

Correct jogging posture. Credit: Kazumi Takeo.

Step by Step

You may have never thought about your cadence, which is the number of steps you take per minute. Well, think about it now: Jog for fifteen seconds around the room, or even in place if you don't have enough space, and count the number of steps (with both feet) that you take.

What's your final number? For beginners it would usually be between thirty-five and forty-four, whereas for professional runners it is on average higher. You got forty-five or more? Congratulations—that's the ideal cadence of 180 steps per minute! If yours was lower, try fifteen seconds of jogging again while consciously aiming at forty-five.

Remembering this rhythm now will come in handy later on. If at some point you get faster and want to participate in a race, you will not need to change your rhythm, just your stride length, or how much ground you cover with each step.

For very low speed, your stride will be very short, about one-third of what you would think of as average running stride. For the speed of two miles per hour, it will mean a single step of almost one feet, and about 1.3 feet for 2.5 miles per hour.

Breathing

During walking or any other physical activity your breathing follows your natural instincts. It's completely automatic, so all you need to do is trust your body.

As running experts, we are often asked about breathing while running. Is it true that it is better to breathe in by your nose and out by your mouth? Even with walking, the oxygen demand increases with speed, which makes you breathe faster and makes your heart beat faster. When you walk slowly, your energy expenditure is three times higher than when sitting still. That figure rises to five times higher for brisk walking and six times when climbing the stairs. Still, in none of the examples above are you consciously controlling the way you breathe. With no effort on your part, your lungs and heart automatically adjust themselves to the activity performed.

The same is true with slow jogging: Trust your instincts, don't push yourself into breathing through your nose, just smile and get going, chatting or singing.

The higher the speed or intensity of exercise, the more oxygen your body needs. Compared to when you're sitting and relaxing, running requires four to five times more oxygen. You can naturally inhale larger volumes of air (and thus oxygen) via your mouth than your nose, but it doesn't mean you need to be particularly conscious about it; your body knows what to do.

There's more to breathing than whether to use your nose or mouth. The amount of oxygen you get depends on the depth of each inhalation as well. Shallow "chest" breathing (marked by your chest rising as you inhale) is much less efficient than deep "belly" breathing (which is marked by your abdomen pushing out as you inhale). If belly breathing doesn't come naturally to you, practice deep inhalation, feeling the air entering your belly. What you feel is actually the diaphragm, the most important breathing muscle. In the act of deep inhalation, you are pushing down into the abdomen to expand the lungs.

Too Busy to Exercise?

We can assure you that in twenty-four hours you will find plenty of occasions to jog, even for a few minutes each time. Contrary to what you may have been told, the effects of interrupted exercise on our health and weight loss are just as promising as continuous exercise.

We particularly recommend slow jogging in the intervals that we mentioned before: One minute of jogging followed by thirty seconds of walking. That's the easiest way to start, particularly recommended for beginners. Try it next time you're walking your dog or on the way to the supermarket—and don't forget about the smile!

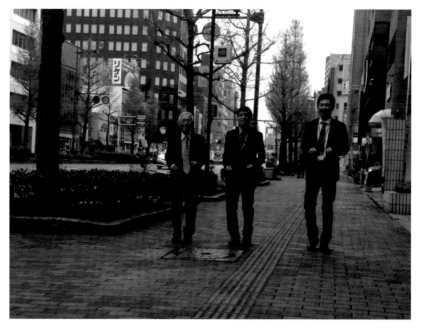

Credit: Magdalena Jackowska

What Do You Need to Start?

Other than some time and willingness to try, you are going to need suitable shoes and clothes.

As we explained above, the right shoes play a crucial role in learning the natural landing technique. Minimalist shoes, sometimes referred to as barefoot shoes, are best. Look for simple shoes with thin, elastic soles and a wide toe box that fit well on the heel.

As for clothing, anything will do as long as it feels comfortable. We've seen slow joggers head to toe in the newest running outfits and businessman on their lunch break jogging in suits.

In summer you want to wear as little clothing as possible. A T-shirt or top and shorts, ideally made of a breathable, quick-drying fabric, are about all you need. Put on running shoes, a cap, a pair of sunglasses, and you are good to go.

In winter you will need a bit more than that, but do not pile on heavy clothing; heavy winter coats are not required. When jogging your body will generate enough heat to keep you warm with a just a wind- and water-resistant jacket. On particularly cold days, a pair of tights and an extra layer of wind-resistant pants should be enough. If you plan to run on the snow or slippery roads you might want to choose trail shoes; otherwise, you will be fine using your regular pair.

All other kinds of running equipment are optional. If it helps you stay motivated, go ahead and invest in a GPS watch. Better yet, reward yourself with a gadget you crave once you reach your target weight or cover your target distance.

The purposes and preferences of slow joggers vary, but *niko niko* is universal. In the next chapter, we'll tell you where the idea came from and, most importantly, how to find your optimal "with a smile" pace.

CHAPTER 4

All About *Niko Niko* Pace

*N*iko niko means "smile" in Japanese. *Niko niko* pace is essentially an easy pace that can be kept with a smile. In this chapter, we'll look in depth at the rationale behind *niko niko* pace, and tell you how to find yours.

As described in Chapter 1, a diagnosis of heart disease led Professor Tanaka to focus on research rather than his own athletic career. Still fond of track and field, he became manager and coach of the university team.

One day during practice he saw an elderly man jogging on the university sports ground, which was quite an unusual sight back then. The man approached young Professor Tanaka and started a conversation.

"You know, I'm going to Germany to participate in World Veteran Sports Championships," the man said. "There is this Olympic coach, Dr. Van Aaken, and he says we should all jog to live a long and happy life until we are 100 years old. Did you know that jogging could prevent you from getting heart disease or cancer? Van Aaken is the one organizing the championships. And his theories are really interesting. Apparently interval training isn't the most optimal method of training; running really slowly is, as it occurs without the accumulation of lactate [a substance produced in human bodies during muscular effort]..."

That elderly man was Hideo Okada, the Japanese record holder for 800 meters. Listening to him, Professor Tanaka remembered that Harald Norpoth, the West German silver medalist at 5,000 meters in the 1964 Tokyo Olympics, has also been also coached by Van Aaken. Tanaka had read an article on Norpoth's training methods and, at the time, was surprised at the low intensity Norpoth recommended. He now believes that having heard about Van Aaken that day must have been fate.

The track and field runners planned their training mostly by themselves, with Tanaka's help. They started analyzing Norpoth's training plans.

In the golden age of interval training, Norpoth—and by extension, Van Aaken—recommended a training method based on long, slow distance, still well known as LSD. He defined LSD as running a long distance at a steady, conversational speed and heart rate below 150 beats per minute (130 beats per minute on average). Van Aaken recommended the same method for almost everyone, from children to the elderly. In 1960, he founded the Western Germany Elderly Long-Distance Runners Association.

It all sparked Professor Tanaka's curiosity about light exercise and became a reason why he started exercising in the "slow" style himself. He hasn't stopped since.

Years later, we have a lot of evidence that light exercise, just as Van Aaken recommended, is effective at both improving athletic performance and simply improving health.

In 1968, Kenneth Cooper's *Aerobics* became a bestseller. Van Aaken, however, recommended lighter exercise than Cooper's exercise prescription. Professor Tanaka knew he wanted to research more in this field. To his great excitement, he was offered a position at Fukuoka University to study exercise prescription under the supervision of a renowned scientist, Professor Shindo.

In the same year, the World Health Organization held a consensus meeting on "Optimal Physical Performance Capacity in Adults." The final paper of this meeting severely underlined the seriousness of hypokinesia, which can lead to the deterioration of the musculoskeletal system and cardiopulmonary functions. It also emphasized the necessity of maintaining a good fitness level to stay healthy. Further, the meeting's eventual findings stressed the importance of training to improve both muscular strength and maximal oxygen uptake (VO2 max). According to the WHO, "From longitude studies it is known that physical training involving large muscle groups that load the oxygen transport system to at least 70–80 percent of the maximal results in an increase in maximal aerobic power." Aerobics as defined by Cooper was also based on exercising at 70–80 percent of VO2 max.

Hideo Okada invited Van Aaken to Japan, and Professor Tanaka was able to learn the training methods from his idol. As it turned out, the base of his theories were in the theses of Wildor Hollman from Germany. Hollman, ex-president of the International Federation of Sports Medicine, was estimating that the lowest optimal exercise intensity was 50 percent of VO2 max, but he didn't conduct any experiments. Together with Professor Shindo, Professor Tanaka and other researchers decided to start the experiments to prove his theories.

The exercise intensity of 50 percent of VO2 max is an extremely interesting intensity from the physiological point of view. That's when the stroke volume of the heart (the volume of blood pumped per one heartbeat) is the largest, lipid metabolism is the highest, and the accumulation of catecholamine (an indicator of lactate and sympathetic nerves' agitation) starts. Catecholamine hardly accumulates until that intensity, but once it's reached, rapid accumulation starts. We hypothesized that at that point, sympathetic nerve activity stimulates training adaptations and improves heart functions without causing significant cardiac stress.

We started studies on a big number of men and women of all ages that revealed a significant increase in their maximal oxygen uptake with physical exercise at the intensity of 50 percent of VO2 max. It is an intensity that we can maintain with a smile, allowing conversation. We called this method training at *niko niko* pace, and started educating people on the concept.

At the same time, we continued studies on the effectiveness of this exercise prescription in hypertension, hyperlipidemia, type-2 diabetes, and cardiac rehabilitation. It led to improvements in all these illnesses and, as we'll see later, in preventing heart disease.

Cooper's *Aerobics* and Bowerman's *Jogging* both were popular guides for beginning American exercisers in the late 1960s. The goal of each was to help people with low fitness progress from walking to being able to run a mile or more. Cooper, for example, recommended starting the first week by walking one mile in 13:30, then gradually adding bouts of running so that by the seventh week the reader was running a mile in a little bit less than 10:00.

That pace probably corresponded to 70 percent of most beginners' VO2 max. Even if it didn't cause them to breathe hard, the effort level was probably considerably hard.

"Slow jogging" at *niko niko* pace, the training method we developed, was significantly lighter. Similarly designed to improve aerobic capacity and health but based on the intensity of just 50 percent of VO2 max, slow jogging means a very relaxed walking pace of 55 yards in 40 to 50 seconds or one mile in 21 to 26 minutes for the least fit runners.

Running in slow jogging style is effective no matter how slow it is. Running one mile you will burn the same number of calories whether your speed is 2 miles per hour or 10 miles per hour. That's why, from the point of view of weight loss, slow jogging pace is equally effective as more strenuous speed. Also, no matter how slow your jogging is, you can burn up to twice the calories you burn walking the same distance.

How to Set Your *Niko Niko* Pace

What do we do when traffic lights are about to turn red? It's one of the moments when even the least fit of us start running. Researches say that, for most of us, this switch from walking to running (known as preferred transition speed) happens at the speed of approximately 4.3 miles per hour, when running becomes a more economical movement than walking. That is also the speed that many of us associate with running, but in our institute we suspected that the comfortable *niko niko* pace for those new to running would be much slower.

In order to prove the validity of this idea, we asked groups of twenty-, fifty-, and seventy-year-old men to run for a couple of minutes at the ultra-slow speed of 1.2 miles per hour. We measured the accumulation of their lactate, to individually estimate how the body reacts to a given volume of exercise. We gradually increased the speed to 2, and later 2.5 miles per hour, in order to observe how their lactate accumulation changed. For those in their twenties, at a speed of around four miles per hour lactate accumulates slightly, similarly to in a resting state, and increases drastically after four miles per hour. For the average fifty-year-old, that moment happened at a speed of three miles per hour, and for seventy-year-olds, at 2.5 miles per hour.

In scientific terms, *niko niko* is the pace that one can keep without significantly exceeding one's lactate threshold, or the point when lactate starts to accumulate dramatically. And that's the pace we recommend for slow jogging, as shown on Professor Tanaka's t-shirt on the next page.

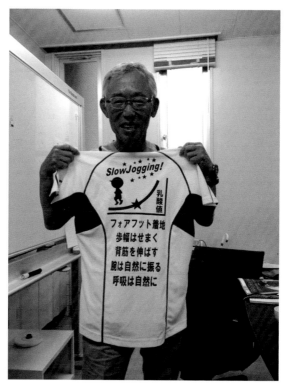

Credit: Sumie Cho

Lactate accumulation measurement allows precision in find-
ing your optimal pace, but for technical reasons not many of you
will have a chance to use it. Fortunately, there are also other, more
accessible methods as well.

Every year, Fukuoka University organizes workshops for amateur runners and marathoners, from teens to those in their seventies or older. During the workshops the participants jog together,
starting at 1.2 miles per hour, and gradually increasing the speed
to 2, 2.5, and 3 miles per hour. After each part we ask the participants to evaluate their fatigue, using the Borg scale that was introduced in Chapter 2.

On this scale of perceived exertion, 6 means rest and 20 is
maximal effort. While repeating short runs at different speeds,

the participants are asked to listen to their bodies, and together we try to estimate what pace will be their optimal slow jogging pace, which is equivalent to an effort level of 10–12 (between "very light" and "light") on the Borg scale. It's best to start with several 1-minute trial runs to find the optimal speed, and at the end try keeping the same pace for 4 minutes to make sure you still feel comfortable. For those with the lowest fitness level, it's usually around 2.5 miles per hour.

Another popular way to estimate exercise intensity is by measuring heart rate. We don't particularly recommend this method, due to big individual differences, but if you want to try, use the following formula: 138 – (your age divided by 2).

If you are thirty, that would be 123 beats/minute, 118 beats/minute for a forty-year-old, 113 beats/minute for a fifty-year-old, and 108 beats/minute for a sixty-year-old. Again, though, it's a formula for beginners, and there can be individual differences of up to 10 to 20 beats per minute. If you're going to estimate *niko niko* pace by heart rate, bear all of this in mind, and if the formula gives you a target heart rate that feels harder than a light effort level, use a lower target heart rate.

No matter what method you choose to estimate it, your optimal pace can be kept with a smile. It's the speed of walking and conversation; if you are out of breath and not able to have a conversation, you should slow. (If you're running alone, you should be able to sing your favorite songs.)

For those of you who are at the beginning of your jogging adventure, *niko niko* pace will probably be lower than walking speed; we suggest starting at 2 to 3 miles per hour. Be warned: It's highly possible that surprised walkers will overtake you. If this happens, just smile and keep going!

CHAPTER 5

How Slow Jogging Improves Your Health and Well-being

Exercise isn't just for elite athletes preparing for competition. With light but regular exercise, everyone can improve their health, fitness, and longevity. Exercise will not only give you a fit and healthy body, but also positive energy, a sense of accomplishment and stress reduction.

In this chapter we'll guide you through the mental and physical health benefits you can experience from slow jogging.

Longevity

Those who exercise tend to be healthier and live longer than those who don't. That's simply a fact that is commonly known and confirmed by numerous studies. What's not as widely known is what dose of exercise gives the highest chance of longevity.

In 2015, Peter Schnohr, MD, of Bispebjerg University Hospital in Denmark announced the results of studies investigating the relation between longevity and pace, quantity, and frequency of jogging, with the joggers divided in groups according to their intensity of exercise. The results suggested that the optimal intensity for jogging is light. Casual joggers were found to have lower mortality rates than more strenuous joggers.

Most of us used to think that the more drained we feel after exercise, the better. Maybe you've skipped exercise altogether, thinking that light workouts are not worth the time. Well, now we know it's not true. The ideal type of exercise for a healthy, long life is . . . slow jogging!

Natural "High"

On some level, we all know that exercise makes us feel better, but we don't usually know why. The beneficial effects of aerobic exercise on anxiety, stress, depression, learning, and aging have all been thoroughly studied by researchers. According to one of the world's specialists in this area, Dr. John Ratey, professor of psychiatry at Harvard Medical School in Boston, "even people who are overweight and who start exercising see improvements in mood and cognition in as little as twelve weeks."

From the 1980s until very recently, endorphins rushing through our body were thought be the main reason for the euphoric emotions during exercise. They are said to trigger a positive feeling, in addition to acting as sedatives and even analgesics, and significantly reduce the perception of pain. Other theories suggested propose that the mood-alternating effects of exercising are possible thanks to increasing serotonin (the neurotransmitter thought to be responsible for feelings of happiness), or brain-derived neurotrophic factor (which supports the growth of neurons).

Only within the last several years has it become clear that the almost miraculous effects of physical activity are mostly due to the endocannabidoid system, responsible for easing our pain, relieving our stress and influencing our mood. In fact, during exercise our body can naturally produce its own version of cannabinoids, such as anandamide, which provide a very similar stimulus to smoking marijuana.

What's particularly interesting is that not all kinds of exercise have the same effect. Studies on runners show that both high-speed running and very low-intensity exercise, such as walking, hardly triggers cannabinoid signaling, whereas the second lowest intensity, defined as "slow jog" produces a drastic increase in their level.

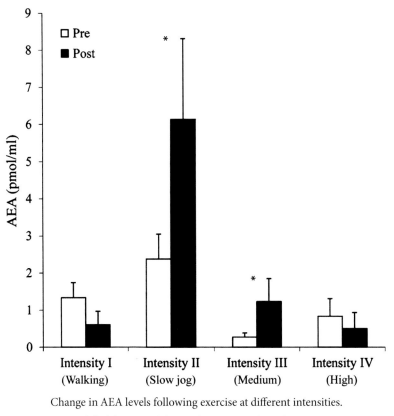

Change in AEA levels following exercise at different intensities.

(Modified from Raichlen et al, 2013). Credit: Yuki Tomiga

To put it simply, slow jogging is perfect in terms of post-exercise effects, including providing a sense of well-being, calm, anxiety, and pain reduction. This also explains the "runner's high," the famous sensation of euphoria of long-distance runners, which has been described as a "feeling of being invincible, a reduced state of discomfort or pain, and even a loss in sense of time while running," as Jesse Pittsley, PhD., from the American Society for Exercise Physiologists states.

Long Life in Good Health

There are various reasons to pick up an exercise habit. When we are young, we usually just want to look fit and make new friends at the gym or jogging path. Later, often in our thirties, we discover that simple daily activities are not always that simple anymore. Running out of breath while climbing the stairs or following our children around the playground often becomes a motivation to get ahold of ourselves. Another ten years down the road it's not just the looks and general fitness anymore. We start having various health issues, and we spend more and more time and money on treatments.

Nearly 75 percent of all deaths in the United States are attributed to the same ten causes, with heart disease remaining as the lead cause; this accounts for one in every four deaths. Not only heart disease, but also the vast majority of "natural" death causes, including stroke, diabetes, and Alzheimer's, are strongly related to our inactive, sedentary lifestyle. Studies show that people who sit still more than four hours per day have a 40 percent higher risk of chronic diseases than those that sit fewer than four hours per day! And while we can't all leave our office desks for the sake of health, we can and should change what we do the rest of the time.

Slow Jogging Comes to the People

Faced with the plague of diseases of affluence, in 1989 the Japanese Health Ministry started to officially encourage physical activity at *niko niko* pace. In 1995, the American College of Sports Medicine also confirmed the effectiveness of light physical activity. Studies in Japan and America continued providing more and more proof for its efficiency in preventing diseases and improving health.

This rapidly increasing popularity led to a TV program on Japanese NHK in 2009, when for the first time slow jogging was shown to a wider public. The reaction was incredible: Phone calls, thankful letters and emails, invitations to lectures and conferences from around the country. Those who had never considered running before felt inspired enough to give it a try. Much to their surprise, they soon felt better and healthier, and found themselves (pleasantly) addicted to slow jogging.

The second big wave of the slow jogging boom came in the fall of 2015. Japanese Empress Michiko appeared on national TV on the day of her eighty-first birthday and explained that she jogs every day to stay in good health. The video featuring Emperor Akihito's and Empress Michiko's slow jogging session appeared on all the main TV stations. Within days there was a visible increase in elderly slow joggers on streets all around the country.

No matter the reason that you first started to exercise, it will definitely influence many aspects of your health to an extent you might not even expect.

Theoretically we all know that exercise is good for health, but what does it actually mean to exercise for health? What kind of exercise are we talking about? And how often?

Almost 2,500 years ago, Hippocrates recommended "give every individual the right amount of exercise, not too little and not too much." That advice remains essential today.

Several decades ago we decided to focus our studies on individually adjusted optimal exercise intensity. It gradually became clear that thirty minutes a day of physical activity light enough to be done with a smile can make miracles happen. Looking for a method that complies with these criteria led to the beginnings of our *niko niko* pace theory and slow jogging.

The method, which is based on *niko niko* pace, was first recommended to Japanese people as early as in 1977, when exercise was associated with competition, sweat, and tears, not pleasure and fun.

Let's now take a look at how slow jogging can help prevent and treat various medical conditions.

Metabolic Syndrome

Metabolic syndrome is not a specific disease itself, but the name for a group of risk factors (that tend to but do not have to occur together) that increase the risk of heart disease and other health problems, such as diabetes and stroke. A person suffering from the metabolic syndrome is twice as likely to develop heart disease and five times as likely to develop diabetes.

As many as 34 percent of American adults have three or more of the following symptoms of metabolic syndrome:

- abdominal obesity
- higher level of triglycerides

- low HDL cholesterol
- high blood pressure
- high blood sugar

The consequences of metabolic syndrome can be life-threatening, but prevention and treatment are based on simple, sustained changes in daily habits.

Slow jogging not only prevents metabolic syndrome, but significantly increases the fitness level, thereby lowering mortality even in those already suffering from the syndrome. The results of our study in Tokyo showed that, in a group of 9,000 office workers, the cancer mortality rate of those of the high fitness level was 59 percent lower compared to those of the lowest fitness level.

High Blood Pressure

How does exercise affect your blood pressure? The right dose of regular physical activity will make your heart stronger, so that it can pump more blood with every beat it takes, with less effort. That means that the stress on arteries gets lower, and so does your blood pressure.

We asked a group of elderly patients (seventy-five years old on average) suffering from heart diseases and high blood pressure to participate in our *niko niko* pace study. They continued to take their medicine during the program; the only change in their lifestyle was introducing thirty minutes to one hour of exercise at *niko niko* pace three to five times a week for three months.

Before the study, the participants had been taking medicine for a long time, so their systolic blood pressure was stable at 140mm Hg, and their diastolic pressure was 80mm Hg. After the study period, their blood pressure was even lower, at an average of 130/70.

The improvement that was not possible with traditional medicine alone, turned out to be achievable with training at *niko niko* pace and allowed the patients to get their results back to norm! What the study also showed was that you need to continue exercising to keep your blood pressure low, so remember to keep working out once you get better.

HDL ("Good Cholesterol")

Cholesterol, which is usually associated with being harmful to your health, can actually be good or bad, depending on its kind. LDL cholesterol is considered the bad one; high levels of it put you at risk of arteriosclerosis and heart disease. On the other hand, the good cholesterol, HDL, helps to reduce the bad one; thus, increasing HDL is more than desirable.

The group of patients suffering from high blood pressure introduced above was also asked to have their cholesterol levels checked. It is known that the level of "good" cholesterol is strongly related to the amount of exercise in everyday life. We wanted to check what kind of changes can be achieved with 180 minutes a week of slow jogging at *niko niko* pace (either thirty minutes six times a week, or one hour three times a week). It turned out that, in addition to blood pressure getting lower, HDL levels got higher, allowing us to kill two birds with one stone.

But be warned: As with the blood pressure results, HDL levels also got worse after one month of abandoning regular slow jogging. Establishing your exercise routine is a great first step, but only sticking to it guarantees lifelong results!

Diabetes

In 2012, 29.1 million Americans, or 9.3 percent of the population, suffered from diabetes. With close to two million new diagnoses every year, it remains the seventh leading cause of death in the United States. Moderate exercise such as slow jogging can lower blood sugar levels, improve insulin sensitivity, and strengthen the heart, making working out great and natural medicine.

If you have recently been diagnosed with type 2 diabetes, you probably haven't exercised in years, and the idea of doing so might seem intimidating. Don't worry—as long as you start slowly, exercise is not only perfectly safe, but highly recommended.

A Diabetes Success Story

Mr. S. was diagnosed with type 2 diabetes at the age of seventy-one. When this happened, he started to go for walks, reduced his portion sizes and joined our *niko niko* classes, all as recommended by his doctor. Ten years have passed since he made those lifestyle changes, and he still exercises at *niko niko* pace at least three hours per week.

When he was diagnosed with diabetes, Mr. S's hemoglobin A1c level was 6.8 percent; below 6.5 percent is the norm. Now that reading is between 4.8 and 5.6 percent. Mr. S. is, of course, pleased with the results. He's so pleased, in fact, that he recommends slow jogging to everyone around him.

Sarcopenia

Sarcopenia is defined as loss of muscle mass and strength associated with aging. It leads to impaired mobility, a higher risk of falls, and eventually an increased risk of mortality.

We are usually told we should be doing some kind of muscle training. You probably know that muscles become weaker and smaller with aging, but did you know that the changes vary by muscle groups?

For example, consider the upper-leg muscles. The hamstring muscles, which are found at the back of the upper legs, do not really change over the years, but the quadriceps, on the front, shrink remarkably. The largest muscles groups, such as the buttocks, abdomen, and dorsal muscles, shrink as well.

Disuse of muscles is the main cause behind their shrinking, which is why hamstring muscles that are used when walking do not suffer. However, the muscle groups that shrink are almost not necessary for walking. The best way to prevent sarcopenia is not any specific muscle training; it's simply achieved by using the big muscle groups in our daily life. Running and jogging require the use of all the muscles that would otherwise shrink, making easy and enjoyable jogging a great way to prevent and recover from sarcopenia. But keep in mind that sarcopenia is mostly a problem of the elderly, and it's therefore very important to choose an optimal dose and kind of exercise, one that will not be too strenuous but still effective enough.

Since the muscles most affected by sarcopenia are the muscles we use when running or jogging, we have checked the effects of slow jogging training at a speed equal to or slower than the usual walking speed in older Japanese. Leg muscle strength and mass both significantly increased during a twelve-week program, suggesting that slow jogging can be a great tool to prevent and cure sarcopenia.

Healthy Body and Healthy Mind

For most of us, the greatest worries related to aging are dementia and aging of the brain. There are two types of dementia: Vascular, which is associated with the aging of the vessels, and Alzheimer's disease, which is associated with changes in the hippocampus, the part of the brain responsible for memory. Most types of dementia are the latter. After the age of seventy, the risk of dementia gets significantly higher, and affects 40 percent of those in their nineties.

Until recently, the decrease in brain cells was thought to be an inevitable consequence of aging, and Alzheimer's was thought to be an incurable disease.

Now we know that the number of brain cells can decrease and increase independently of age. A study on the risk of the disease over a forty-year span on 8,000 inhabitants of the Japanese town of Hisayama showed that those of higher fitness level were at lower risk of Alzheimer's disease.

Another experiment conducted in recent years analyzed the relation between a distance run and the impression of a gene responsible for the increase of hippocampus cells. The mice in this study were divided in two groups: Running and not-running. Both brain function and the number of hippocampus cells were higher in the running group.

According to one hypothesis, Alzheimer's disease is caused by the accumulation of beta amyloid, a harmful protein in the cells of the hippocampus, resulting in their decay. Studies on mice showed that running helped to stop the amyloid beta synthesis and to keep a constant number of cells.

Until recently it was very difficult to experiment on humans, but now, thanks to MRIs, we can measure brain volume and estimate the relation between fitness level and hippocampus volume and space orientation in the elderly. Specialist in brain-aging and cognitive function, Kirk Erickson, PhD of the University of Pittsburgh, found that the volume of hippocampus is positively related to the aerobic capacity (VO2 max) and can be improved with aerobic training. For this study, 120 participants were divided into two groups: Performing aerobic exercise (walking a gradually increased distance) and stretching, in weekly sessions for one year.

Interestingly, there were significant individual differences between the participants, and the hippocampus volume increased primarily in those whose VO2 max also increased (10 percent or more). Lack of increase or decrease in VO2 max was related to lack of increase or decrease in the hippocampus volume. We can deduce, therefore, that the improvement in VO2 max was vital for the changes in the hippocampus volume. Our studies show that slow jogging is one of the simplest and safest ways to achieve it.

Successive studies featured two groups of young adults (twenty-seven years old on average): Those who slow jogged thirty minutes, three times a week, for twelve weeks, and those leading their regular lives with no changes. The subjects underwent regular measurements to check the functions of their frontal lobe, such as logical thinking, memory, or planning. Before the experiment, the average score in both groups was 70 points (out of a possible 100). In the slow jogging group, the score gradually increased, and was close to 100 by the twelfth week. Slow jogging improved frontal lobe function and thus the whole brain.

A dose of slow jogging every day is a natural method to improve brain and "memory fitness." The sooner you start, the better, even if you are far from being elderly.

Stretching is Not Enough

What kind of exercise can prevent or slow decrease in hippocampus volume? In one study, sixty- and seventy-year-olds were divided into two groups: Brisk walking and stretching. After six months of one hour of the given exercise three times a week, the hippocampus volume for those in the walking group increased, physiologically rejuvenating the subjects. In the stretching group, no changes were observed, suggesting that aerobic exercise is the most beneficial type for brain health.

Common Denominator: Obesity

Most of the health problems described here are directly or indirectly related to obesity. It's not only a problem of aesthetics, but is also a huge factor in most serious diseases. A big project conducted over twenty years in the United States, Australia, and Sweden showed that serious obesity dramatically shortens life—on average, by six-and-a-half years for BMI over 40 and by fourteen years for BMI 55 or higher. Unfortunately, US health officials reported in late 2015 that, despite all the attention given the issue, the percentage of obese Americans has continued to increase.

In the next chapter, we'll see how slow jogging is a fantastic tool for weight loss, regardless of how many pounds you hope to shed.

CHAPTER **6**

Weight Loss with Slow Jogging

Weight loss is among the top reasons to exercise. Unless you're one of the rare few who are naturally skinny well into adulthood, you've probably tried various diets or exercise regimes in the hope of slimming down.

Although we often know what to do in theory to stay in shape, in practice it's not all that simple. Adding to the challenge is that it's easy to believe in the new methods, techniques and machines endlessly touted as making weight loss easier, from vibrating belts to sports games such as WiiFit.

But despite what purveyors of weight-loss "miracles" would like you like to believe, changes in body weight occur in a very simple way: It's all about the balance of calories consumed versus calories expended. Negative balance results in losing weight, whereas positive balance means gaining weight.

Safe, Effective Weight Loss with Slow Jogging

If your goal is sustainable weight loss, a safe but effective target is to burn an extra 300 calories a day. For somebody who weighs 200 pounds, that's the equivalent of, all else being equal, a daily walk of more than four miles. Slow jogging is even more effective at increasing your energy expenditure, and helps you burn up to twice the calories you do when walking. Just a 2.5-mile jog is enough to burn the same 300 calories. That's because when jogging you use the biggest muscle groups in your body—the quadriceps, psoas, and glutes, which are barely used when walking.

It's easy to calculate the energy expenditure for running or jogging. Research has shown that the calories burned while running a given distance are the same, whether that distance is covered by sprinting or slow jogging. The formula is this: Calories burned equal your bodyweight in kilograms per kilometer. Just multiply your daily distance by your weight in kilograms to find the calories burned. For a 200-pound (90 kilogram) person, 2.5 miles (4 kilometers) of slow jogging means an expenditure of 360 calories (90 kilograms X four kilometers). To lose one pound of fat, you need to burn 3,500 kilocalories, so 2.5 miles of slow jogging every day will help you lose your first pound after ten days.

Remember, you can jog just a bit at a time, a couple times a day, whenever you have time. For example, if you jog at three miles per hour, fifty minutes a day, in segments of whatever short length, will give you a total distance of 2.5 miles. This is a great way to get to your daily target when your schedule is extraordinarily busy.

But your perfect body shape is not just the number on the scale, but also body proportions. For most of us, the waist is the most problematic area; that's where vicious fat accumulates first and often to the greatest extent. Good news: With slow jogging, waist fat is easier to get rid of than you'd think. Looking at average changes in waistline and body weight, every pound lost with slow jogging results in almost one inch less around the waist.

Slow Jogging and Diet

That said, if you want slow jogging to help you lose weight, you'll need to pay attention to what you eat as well. Consider a study conducted on the changes in appetite in mice exercising various amounts of time per day. For those in the study running one to five hours a day, the more they exercised, the more they ate. These participants were allowed to eat as much as they wanted to, so in the group that exercised the most, the intake of calories was always the highest. Despite all the exercise, their weight remained the same. If you just trust your gut, so to speak, the same will probably happen to you—the more you run, the bigger your appetite will be, and you might not shed the extra pounds.

Interestingly, the mice that exercised less than one hour a day had a tendency to eat more calories than they burned, and their body weight increased. If losing weight is your main goal, you should be careful about your food choices. Small doses of exercise should not become an excuse to unlimited consumption. Weight loss is much faster and safer when you combine exercise with mild calorie restrictions. A study we conducted provides support for this approach.

We asked a group of sedentary patients suffering from a metabolic syndrome to participate in our study comparing different ways of weight reduction, and divided them into three groups: Exercise only, diet (calorie restriction) only, and exercise and diet combined. Let's take a look at the results.

Exercise Only: The participants, who all had no habit of any sort of regular exercise before the experiment, were asked to exercise at *niko niko* pace for a total of 300 minutes (five hours) a week or more. Once a week, they came to the university for an exercise session together (slow jogging, cycling and step exercise, all at their prescribed *niko niko* pace). On other days, they did slow jogging by themselves. After three months, the average weight loss in this group was four-and-a-half pounds.

Based on this study (and numerous others performed around the world), if you're not particularly impatient about your weight loss, it will be enough to just add some exercise (we recommend slow jogging) to your everyday routine. As we saw earlier, a 200-pound person slow jogging two-a-half miles per day will burn more than an extra 300 calories daily, which will lead to a loss of one pound after ten days. But remember: Covering the same distance walking instead of slow jogging will result in only about 170 calories burned per day. Slow jogging can double the energy expenditure of walking.

Also remember that you don't have to cover your daily distance all at once. You might have heard that short bouts of exercise burn only carbohydrates, not fat, and thus aren't effective in weight loss. This isn't the case—no matter what fuels our body during exercise, the extra energy consumption will lead to negative calorie balance and thus weight loss. Two and a half miles of jogging, broken into short periods and spread out during the day, is possible even with the busiest schedules. Try the intermittent slow jogging for twenty minutes in the morning (combination of one minute of jogging and thirty seconds of walking), twenty minutes before lunch, and another twenty minutes before dinner. Try also to fit even shorter cycles any time during the day, such as on the way to the bathroom or shopping. In one study we conducted, a group who followed something like this approach lost an average of six pounds in three months, without consciously altering their eating habits. As in the mice study above, it turned out that this moderate amount of exercise didn't result in them having more of an appetite.

<u>Diet Only</u>: The second group in our experiment was on a calorie restriction program, without exercise. Their individual, optimal calorie intake was calculated on the basis of their ideal body mass index. Once a week, they consulted a university dietician.

The significant reduction in calorie consumption resulted in an average loss of seven pounds in three months. Similar to the exercise group, they experienced health benefits associated with weight loss such as increased insulin sensitivity, but the downside was their muscle mass loss. Both their aerobic capacity and "good" cholesterol level didn't change.

<u>Exercise and Diet</u>: The third group followed the exercise recommendations given to the first group and the calorie restrictions of the second group. After three months, they lost an average of almost nine pounds, without losing muscle mass, while increasing their aerobic capacity and "good" cholesterol level, making it by far the most beneficial method of the three.

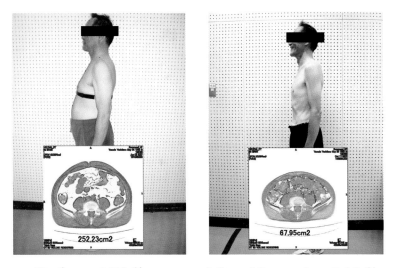

Before: 176 lbs.   After 12 weeks: 145 lbs.

A participant in the Exercise and Diet group before and after the experiment.

Credit: Hiroaki Tanaka, Magdalena Jackowska

Never Yo-Yo Diet Again

If you drastically reduce your calorie intake, you'll lose weight. But, as many people know too well, maintaining the lighter weight can be much more challenging than dieting itself. Extreme diets, in particular those excluding whole food groups, will inevitably make you lose muscle tissue and slow your basal metabolism.

The more muscle you have, the more calories your body burns even when you're not working out, so even if you're not interested in looking like a body builder, muscle loss is something you definitely want to avoid.

Frustrating as it is, not only post-diet overeating, but even simply returning to your pre-diet eating habits, especially if you lost muscle tissue, will guarantee weight regain and maybe even some extra new pounds.

Those irritating side effects of dieting are avoidable if you combine a reasonable calorie restriction with easy exercise, such as slow jogging. The key to success is to keep exercising, even after you achieve your weight goal. Eat normally but choose smaller portions on days when you can't work out. That's pretty much enough to keep you yo-yo-free forever!

Calories In, Calories Out

The recommended daily amount of calories for adults according to US dietary guidelines is around 2,000. That figure isn't correct for everyone and depends on your lifestyle, but for now let's use it as reference. We know that a daily 30 percent reduction of consumed calories, leaving us with 1,400 calories, is not only safe, but shown to help longevity (proven to be associated with expression of sirtuin genes, known as longevity genes). As you remember, we need to burn 3,500 calories to lose one pound. So a daily reduction of 600 calories will help you lose one pound in about six days.

> However, if you introduce some exercise to your daily schedule, with the same amount of calories consumed, you can lose fat much faster.

Even 2.5 miles of slow jogging every day adds another 300 calories to your deficit, meaning that now you're burning an extra 900 calories a day (600 from your food intake and 300 from slow jogging), and will lose a pound in just four days.

Of course, adding slow jogging to your plan isn't only about burning more calories. It will also stop your metabolism from slowing down, which very often becomes a reason of rapid weight gain after achieving your target. And because the 300 calories from slow jogging can be accumulated during the whole day, even those with a busy schedule should be able to do it.

If you have more time or more weight to lose, you can try to exercise even more. Especially at the beginning of dieting, losing weight quickly can help to mentally set you on the right track and keep you motivated.

Eating Habits

While there are numerous detailed menu plans available on the market, thinking of some manageable changes in your current eating habits is probably a better place to start.

Depending on your lifestyle and diet targets, there may be various ways to achieve your goal, but a golden rule we recommend to every beginner is to reduce the amount of consumed carbohydrates and fat while increasing the amount of protein. This can be done primarily with some easy changes in the products you use and how you cook.

For example, if you're addicted to fast-food hamburgers, try tricking your brain by eating a sub, but one that is filled with lean meats instead. If you can't imagine your life without starches, choose grains, potatoes, and everything whole-wheat rather than white bread. Prepare your meals by grilling, boiling, or steaming instead of frying. Use dressing based on vinegar, soy sauce, or lemon instead of artificial ones full of fat and sugar. The list can go on and on. We also encourage you to do your own research. First-hand experience will teach you more than theory.

Be careful with animal sources of protein, as they can also contain a lot of fat. Choose lean proteins such as beef, pork, and chicken. A good solution is fish, which is high in protein and low in fat (and that's mostly the more healthful non-saturated fat). White fish, tuna, squid, shrimp, octopus, and shellfish all contain about 100 calories per 100 grams, including about 20 grams of protein. Vegetarians and vegans have plenty of beans and legumes to choose from.

So, what can we suggest for your main meals? Begin with the Japanese approach to meal preparation. Focus on quality over quantity and, whenever possible, choose food that's fresh, seasonal, local, and minimally processed.

To start the day, there is nothing we can recommend more than a green smoothie. For a satisfying, but low-calorie option, try our favorite:

- a handful of green leafy vegetables (spinach, kale, etc.)
- half an ounce of avocado
- half a banana
- two ounces of plain yogurt
- 1/3 cup milk

Mix all the above and blend until smooth to get a 150- to 200-calorie morning meal that's full of fiber, vitamin, and minerals, and will keep you going for hours.

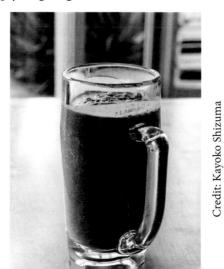

Credit: Kayoko Shizuma

For many of us, there's not much time to think about lunch. If that's the case with you, pick up a take-out meal that features lean, healthful ingredients. You're likely to get a bigger portion than you need. Eat half, and save the other half for the following day.

Dinner? Now it's time to enjoy life and reward yourself for all the hard work! As long as you don't overdo your portions and stick to your slow jogging routine, you should still be able to keep a daily negative calorie balance.

Maintaining Balance

When deciding on a weight-loss program, focus on your lifestyle and what's doable for you. You'll need to make changes that will work for months or years, rather than days or weeks.

Equally important, you'll need to make changes that won't stop you from enjoying life. We all have our habits and small pleasures that we won't be able to (or want to) give up on permanently. For many Japanese, that means a late-night meal washed down with beer, as a way to relax and provide a mental boost after a long, stressful work day.

Now, we're not suggesting that you should feel good about late-night overeating or drinking. But we want to you to understand that, in the long run, adjusting eating habits to fit your lifestyle and sticking to them will be much more important than what particular menu or diet you choose to follow.

Common sense and energy balance is the key to success. Instead of avoiding all your guilty pleasures, include them in your menu and plan the rest of it accordingly. If you sometimes go overboard, go for a longer jog or be careful the following day to neutralize the effects of your "debauchery."

Keep Calm and Carry On

We've all been there: It's the morning after a dinner party, you get on the scale and see that you've put on several pounds, and you start panicking. This frequent scenario can easily discourage impatient dieters.

Relax! To really put on three pounds of fat, you would need to consume more than 10,000 extra calories. Considering that we consume on average 2,000 to 3,000 calories daily, taking in 10,000 is almost impossible. (Ever tried eating forty-five chocolate bars in one sitting?) The sudden weight increase following a dinner party is mostly due to water retention, which is temporary.

Instead of thinking in terms of every meal, it's more realistic to count total calories in one day or even a couple of days. The same applies to what you see on the scale—what matters is the pattern over time, not any one isolated reading. Again, enjoy your new lifestyle so that you're able to continue it for a long time.

Professor Tanaka's Weight-Loss Challenge

Professor Tanaka overcame obesity and metabolic syndrome in 1994, and has been slim ever since. Here's what he did in his first few months of his new lifestyle.

Because he was so busy during the day, he found it easier to reduce his caloric intake in the morning and/or at lunch. At breakfast, he started to avoid butter or had one fewer piece of toast. At lunch, he chose something satisfying but low in calories, like buckwheat noodles (soba). If he had a bento box with large portions, he left part of it. He didn't cut out desserts, as he finds them to be small, but important everyday pleasures. He chose ones low in calories, or ate a smaller portion of richer desserts.

As far as exercise is concerned, he was aiming at burning 300 to 400 calories a day, which in his case meant covering about four miles by slow jogging. He would usually jog for thirty minutes in the morning and add the remaining miles before lunch or dinner.

The results of his challenge are shown below:

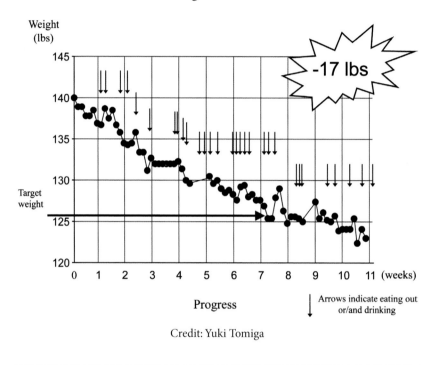

Credit: Yuki Tomiga

Japanese Cuisine: A Diet Without a Diet

The Japanese pride themselves on being one of the healthiest nations in the developed world. Japanese women returned to the top of world longevity rankings in 2012; their average lifespan is 86.61 years. Japanese men rank fourth on the longevity list, with an average of 80.21 years.

At the same time, the obesity rate is one of the lowest, with only 3.5 percent of the population classified as obese, compared to rates as high as 30 percent or more in countries like the United States.

And while genetics and a generally healthy lifestyle do play a role, an undeniable part of the well-being is rooted in the eating habits.

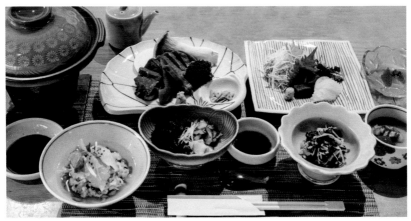

Credit: Kayoko Shizuma

The growing popularity of Japanese cuisine and its availability make it more and more common around the world. International appreciation for Japanese cuisine was confirmed in 2013, when it was added to UNESCO's Intangible Cultural Heritage list. But Japanese food is not only sushi and green tea; it's history, culture, and love of food.

Japanese cuisine, as certified by UNESCO, is based on four principles:

<u>Ingredients</u>: Those crucial in Japan are mostly rice, fish and seafood, seaweed and vegetables. Equally important is variety, quality, respect for nature, minimal processing, and modest use of spices.

Composition: 1 + 1 + 2, where rice is served with soup, such as miso soup (1); a main dish, usually fish (1); and two side dishes, usually vegetables or tofu (2).

Nutritional Values: The typical proportions of macro-nutrients are 13 percent protein, 25.5 percent fat, and 61.5 percent carbohydrates.

Ritual: The key words here are flavor, pleasure, and celebration, but also *savoir-vivre* and appreciation of food. Traditionally, the dishes are consumed at the same time, with neutral rice eaten in between more intense dishes.

Japanese food, even without particular calorie restrictions, can be beneficial for a healthy diet and even weight loss. It's not only the ingredients, but the approach to and the culture of food that's something we can learn from.

CHAPTER 7
Self-Care and Injury Prevention

Someone once said that running a marathon, which is 42 kilometers long, is not such a big deal, and that the real challenge is to keep running and enjoying it for forty-two years. We couldn't agree more. There's not only the matter of staying motivated for many years, but also of staying healthy and injury-free. In this chapter, we'll see the many things you can do to take care of yourself so that you can enjoy a lifetime of slow running.

Avoiding injuries is essential for every runner who hopes to have a long running career. The first and most essential point here is learning the correct and natural running technique. Make sure you read and understood the forefoot landing theory we described in Chapter 3.

As with most kinds of physical activity, running is easier if you warm up a bit beforehand. Slow jogging is a very gentle form of exercise, so it's enough to stretch the main muscles in your legs, start walking, and proceed to jogging. If you are planning on a more intense training, slow jogging itself is a great warm-up.

The risk of injuries is greater when you run fast or long distances. Listen to both your body and your common sense. When you do run a longer distance, divide it in smaller parts and break your run down. For beginners, that would mean sections of ten minutes; for veterans, around thirty minutes. Complete beginners can alternate one minute of jogging and thirty seconds of walking.

Be Careful with Hard Interval Training

Many ambitious runners tend to believe that the more exhausted they feel after training, the more effective it is.

Interval training first gained popularity thanks to the Czechoslovakian runner Emil Zátopek, who won a total of five medals—four of which were golds—in the 1948 and 1952 Olympics. While it can be a powerful method for runners aiming to improve their results in track races, interval training is not really necessary if you're preparing for a marathon, and is certainly not integral to running for health, general fitness, and weight loss. In addition, if you overdo interval training, the fatigue becomes cumulative, making it a lot easier to overtrain and get injured. Slow jogging and intervals at *niko niko* pace can give you sufficient results without the pain.

Crosstraining and Step Exercise

Any exercise that places continuous, repeated stress on the same parts of the body can lead to injuries. That's why crosstraining is a great idea. Instead of just jogging or running, supplement it with walking, cycling, or swimming. Cycling and swimming are perfect to improve your stamina and performance.

There's another method of crosstraining we recommend that's equally effective and even more accessible than cycling or swimming. It's step exercise, which is ideal when the time of day or weather are making it difficult to enjoy a jog outside. Step exercise also improves your running because it builds stability in your ankles. Thirty minutes of step exercise during one part of the day and thirty minutes of slow jogging at another time of day is a great combination.

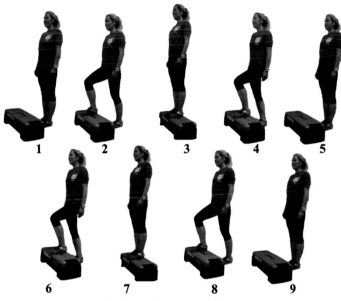

Credit: Kazumi Takeo, Yoichi Hatamoto

You can use anything as your step: a seat, bench or even a box filled with old magazines. The exercise couldn't be simpler. Start with your right leg and climb the step, follow with your left leg, and get down with your right leg first and then left. Make sure to straighten your knees when on the top of the step. If you're injured or elderly, you can use a rail for support.

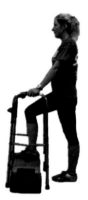

Credit: Kazumi Takeo, Yoichi Hatamoto

Beginners can start with ten sets of going up and down per minute on a step of around eight inches, which is the average height of stairs. That's the equivalent of jogging at 1.2 miles per hour.

You can easily adjust the exercise intensity by going a bit faster, with these equivalencies:

15 up-and-down sets per minute give you exercise similar to around 2 miles per hour.

20 sets per minute is roughly equal to 2.5 miles per hour.

25 sets per minute is roughly equal to 3 miles per hour.

30 sets per minute is roughly equal to 4 miles per hour.

If You Get Injured

Even with perfect running technique and self-care, injuries can occur, sometimes as a result of training, sometimes not.

When you can't exercise due to injury, you have to be careful about not putting on weight. Naturally if we train less than usual but still eat to satisfy our appetite, it's easy to take in too many calories. Pay attention to your diet and the ingredients of your meals. While you're injured, stay motivated to monitor your weight by telling yourself that extra weight could lead to reinjury when you're able to start training again.

There are many ways to exercise that avoid working the injured section of your body too much. For example, if your knee hurts, try cycling or swimming, which don't put so much stress on your knee. Both will help to keep your heart and lungs fit, and will help you avoid weight gain.

The step exercise that we described above is also a great alternative training. That's actually how the method first gained popularity: We recommended it to Harumi Yanagawa, a blind runner who was the gold medalist in the marathon at the 1996 Paralympics. Even with the typical injuries like runner's knee, the step exercise in moderation is still possible, as long as you don't feel pain. Thanks to the method, Yanagawa was able to keep training and finished the race with a great time. Since then we have seen numerous runners who were not able to continue their regular training due to injuries but stayed in good shape for the race. Sometimes they even improved their results using step exercise as an alternative training method.

Take a Break

Pain can, and often should, be interpreted as a warning from your body, so if something really hurts, just take a break. Think of it as a chance to recover physically and mentally. Although some people believe that, after one week without exercise, it takes one month to return to your previous shape, there's no scientific data to support that belief.

Take a look at the graph below, showing the changes in Professor Tanaka's maximal oxygen uptake over the years. It shows his maximum oxygen consumption at the age of thirty-two and its

value fourteen years later, before he started training on a regular
basis.

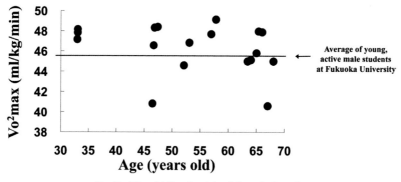

Credit: Hiroaki Tanaka, Magdalena Jackowska

Sure enough, due to aging and lack of exercise, this value
became lower. Still, very soon after Professor Tanaka started training again, it got back to a level similar to what it was at in his
younger days. It was lower again at the time when he was injured
and couldn't train, but after resuming regular exercise, after two
months it was again at the same level that it was twenty-two years
before.

At age sixty-three, Professor Tanaka broke bones in his shoul-
der and upper arm while skiing. He was unable to run for several
months, and once again his VO2 max decreased sharply. Several
months after he recovered and resumed slow jogging, he was back
again at the same fitness level. Similarly, however long your break
from exercising may be, you can recover considerably quickly.
We have heard of many examples of runners who kept running
despite injuries and got gradually worse. When it hurts, be smart
enough to stop training.

Meridian Test

The Meridian Test (also known as M-Test), one of the most popular methods of sports medicine in Japan, was developed by a friend, Dr. Yoshito Mukaino, who is a renowned physician and fellow professor at Fukuoka University. The M-Test is a holistic diagnostic tool based on the meridian system of acupuncture. It gained worldwide popularity as a powerful treatment and self-care method, and is used to improve athletic performance and physical fitness.

The goal, according to Professor Mukaino, is to identify movements that cause or aggravate pain or inhibit range of motion, which in turn indicates which meridians should be treated. It consists of simple stretches of the whole body, as shown below.

Upper-body Stretches

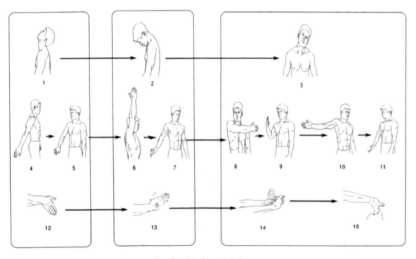

Credit: Yoshito Mukaino

Lower-body Stretches

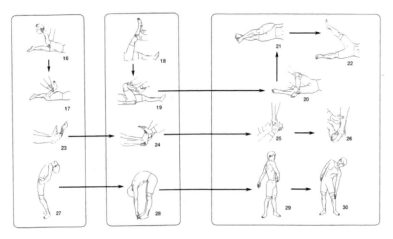

Credit: Yoshito Mukaino

Neck Stretches

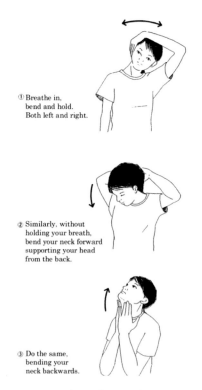

① Breathe in,
bend and hold.
Both left and right.

② Similarly, without
holding your breath,
bend your neck forward
supporting your head
from the back.

③ Do the same,
bending your
neck backwards.

Credit: Yoshito Mukaino

Daily stretches before and after training will help make your body more flexible and prevent injuries. Stretching the opposite part of the body to the one that feels strained is very effective. If the pain doesn't go away, it might mean that there is a more serious organic problem and you should look for professional orthopedic help.

For more details, check out Professor Mukaino's book *Sports Acupuncture: The Meridian Test and Its Applications* (Eastland Press, 2008) and website (www.mtestusa.com).

Daily Habits, Rules to Remember

Theoretically, we all know that it's easier to prevent injuries than treat them. But in our busy everyday lives, it's hard to put that knowledge into practice, often until it's too late. A few good habits, however, can go a long way toward keeping your body healthy enough to hold up to your training. Try to make these simple practices part of your life:

- Listen to your body and common sense.
- Don't overdo it.
- Allow yourself enough rest and enough sleep.
- Stretch regularly using the M-Test.
- Get relaxing baths and a massage every now and then.
- After harder training, ice your tendons and muscles. Massage the tense places while taking a bath.
- Maintain your optimal body weight.
- Refer to the tips on diet in Chapter 6.

Your body will thank you and reward you with years of enjoyable exercise.

CHAPTER 8

Slow Jogging and Your First Marathon

So you've been running regularly for a while, can keep a steady pace for an hour or longer, and enjoy yourself doing so. Is it time to take on the most hallowed of races, the marathon? Should you do so even if you've never run a race?

While there's nothing wrong with running a marathon as your first race (if you're adequately prepared), you might want to start with a 5K (3.1 miles) or 10K (6.2 miles), and gradually build up from there. There are many fun opportunities to enjoy your first race experience at a shorter distance without the competitive atmosphere.

Further, races at distances shorter than the marathon, including the half marathon, are in many ways similar to your regular training and to some extent predictable. Yes, you run with a crowd and experience all the emotions of a race, but the running part itself will probably not involve anything you haven't experienced.

Beyond the half marathon, and especially after twenty miles, things become more unpredictable, as your body reacts to efforts it has never experienced before. Even if it's not your first one, every marathon is different; maybe it's the thrill of the unknown that makes us want to try again and again.

Let's look at what you need to know before tackling your first marathon.

A Brief History of the Marathon

It all started in ancient Greece in 490 B.C. After a crushing victory by the Greeks over the Persians, Pheidippides set on a journey to bring the good news to Athens. According to the legend, he ran more than forty kilometers from the battlefield in Marathon to Athens to deliver the happy message. "*Niki!*" ["Victory!"] he shouted, and died, exhausted.

His heroic run was commemorated in the first modern Olympic Games in 1896 in Greece with a forty-kilometer run from Marathon Bridge to the Olympic Stadium in Athens. A Greek postal worker, Spiridon Louis, won in 2:58:50.

The current marathon distance is slightly longer. In 1908, Queen Aleksandra requested that the marathon race during the London Olympics start on the lawn of Windsor Castle and finish in front of the royal box at the Olympic Stadium. That's when the distance changed to 26.2 miles (42.2 kilometers). Since the 1924 Olympics in Paris, the marathon has been standardized at that distance.

The Marathon by the Numbers

We've come a long way since 1896, when nine runners finished the first marathon.

John McDermott, winner of the first Boston Marathon in 1897, completed the old course (24.5 miles) in 2:55:10. In 1926 in London, Violet Percy became the first woman to officially finish a marathon; she ran 3:40:22. In 1953, Jim Peters ran the first sub-2:20 (2:18:40), and fourteen years later Derek Clayton became the first to break 2:10 (2:09:36). The year 1971 was critical for female runners: Elizabeth Bonner ran the first women's sub-3:00 (2:55:22), and three months later Cheryl Bridges ran the first sub-2:50 (2:49:40).

Frank Shorter's Olympic victory in 1972 inspired the American running boom. There are now more than five hundred thousand finishers just in US marathons each year, and hundreds of thousands in other countries. These days, marathons are no longer the domain of young and fast runners. The average finishing time gets slower every year, and almost half of marathoners are age forty or older.

Marathons Around the World

Now you can run marathons in practically every corner of the world, including such extremes as the Sahara Desert, Antarctica, or the Great Wall in China. Of the world's fifteen largest marathons, seven are held in the United States, five in Japan, and three in Europe.

You can also find marathons of all sizes, from local events with a handful of runners on up to the New York City Marathon, the world's largest, which has more than fifty thousand finishers. Many marathons would be even larger if everyone who wanted to run them did. For example, Japan's largest, the Tokyo Marathon, has "only" thirty-five thousand participants, but more than 300,000 people apply for those limited spots every year.

Are You Ready?

Completing a marathon is never easy. It's obviously not easy for those running for the first time, but trust us, it's also not easy for experienced runners either. Still, there must be a reason why hundreds of thousands of people tackle the distance every year.

It's not easy but it can become easier, enjoyable, and even addictive. It can give you a sense of accomplishment that goes far beyond your running life and boosts your confidence in all other aspects.

Marathon running is probably one of the few activities that, in the space of a few hours, will make you experience so much pain and excitement, desperation and joy. You're going to hate yourself and feel proud, and doubt everything but eventually feel more confident than ever. Maybe the overwhelming hopelessness and emotions will even make you cry. But somehow, minutes after finishing the race, still sweaty and sore, you'll find yourself thinking about the next chance to do it again.

Having said that, we're not here to tell you that everyone should run a marathon. That's especially true if you don't feel ready to do it. But if you've been following our advice on the general principles of slow jogging and feel tempted to try a marathon, why not do it? Although you may regret it on the way, you won't once you cross the finish line.

Just choose it, plan it, and run it wisely.

And remember that you don't have to finish at all costs. Sure, you don't want to give up in your first marathon, but if you're really injured, it's better to withdraw and try again when you're healthy. There will be plenty of marathons to choose from when your body and mind are up for the challenge.

Setting a Goal Time

Choosing the right pace is difficult for all marathoners, but particularly so for first-timers. If you trust your intuition and run at the pace that feels just right, it's quite likely that, overwhelmed with emotions, you'll go too fast in the first half and suffer in the second.

We recommend using the Borg scale of perceived exertion that we introduced in Chapter 2. *Niko niko* pace usually corresponds to 10–12 on the scale; consciously trying to stay at that relaxed effort should help you to avoid running too fast too soon. Just be careful—races make us all excited, and when running with a crowd it's easy to start far beyond your comfortable pace without realizing you're doing so until it's too late.

In your first marathon, run at that steady pace of 10–12 on the Borg scale throughout. At the very end, if you feel you still have some energy left, you can always speed up for the last mile or two.

If you want to set a more specific time goal, you can estimate it from times at shorter races. Dr. Tim Noakes, author of *Lore of Running*, suggests multiplying your best half marathon time by 2.11 to get a target marathon time. To use a 10K time, Noakes suggests multiplying that time by 5.5 and subtracting twenty-eight minutes.

If you don't think you can run the whole way, choose a marathon with a time limit of at least seven hours and cover it with a combination of jogging and walking.

One Month Before the Marathon

One month or at least the last three weeks before the race is the time to relax, known among marathon runners as "tapering."

Many of us, especially beginners, feel anxious with the day of the marathon approaching and tend to train harder and harder in the last weeks or even days before the race. We definitely don't recommend this strategy.

Soon before the race is the time to repair the muscle damages and fatigue accumulated during months of training. During this time, you want to reduce the odds of getting injured as much as possible. If you haven't trained enough for the marathon, making up for it at the very last minute isn't going to help, and might make things worse. Start the last month with your regular training plan and gradually decrease the intensity and distance to finish with no running in the last few days.

Take extra steps to avoid injury during this time. We mean not only the obvious injuries, such as torn muscles, but also micro-damages that accumulate without you even realizing. This kind of injury occurs particularly often with eccentric muscle contractions during high-speed training or downhill running. During the last month before the marathon, choose flatter courses and focus your training on slow jogging.

Running less in the last week before the race is not only about physiology; it's also important psychologically. After months of training on a regular basis, you may feel unnatural running much less than usual in the last weeks and close to nothing in the last days before the race. That's exactly the way you should feel when you stand there waiting for the marathon to start—a hunger for running is the best state of mind you can hope for.

The week before the marathon is crucial. It's your final chance to recover from any remaining fatigue, get enough sleep and provide your body with all the necessary nutrients to carry you over 26.2 miles. During this week your meals, rather than your training, have the biggest influence on your race-day performance. Don't experiment with anything you haven't tried so far, in terms of both meals and training.

What to Eat?

You might have already heard of glycogen loading or carbo-loading. While it's not something you necessarily need to try before your first marathon, it's worth knowing about and doing at some point in your marathon career.

As we saw in Chapter 6, the most accessible source of energy for running is glycogen, the carbohydrates and glucose stored in your muscles. It works like gasoline—the more glycogen you store, the farther you can go. The capacity to store glycogen is limited, but research has found that certain food choices and meal strategies in the week before the race can help you store up to double the regular amount of glycogen. For your first marathon, our glycogen-loading recommendation is simple.

Start one week before the race, which will most likely be on a Sunday. First, you want to use up the glycogen stored in your body. To do that, go for a longer jog, preferably twice your usual distance, one week before race day. You can but don't have to eat less carbohydrates in the following three days. During that time, train in the same way you always do, but stop for the last three days before the race. If your race is on Sunday, your last training should be on Wednesday; you can run up to double your regular distance on that day. If you really want to, you can jog in the last three days, but keep the intensity very low and the distance short.

In the last few days before the marathon, load up on glycogen; the simpler, the better. The best examples of carbohydrates to eat now are bread, pasta, rice, cereal, potatoes, Japanese rice cakes (mochi), and fruit. Be careful about high-fiber foods close to the race. They are slower to digest and can cause bloating and gas. The day before the race, avoid eating lots of vegetables and beans, as well as foods that have added fiber, such as high-fiber or bran cereals. Eating sweets and cakes is fine, as long as they're not high in fat. Most of the calories you eat during this time should come from carbohydrates, not fat or protein.

Other Pre-Race Matters

Choosing your target pace and effective carbo-loading are your priority before the race, but you can increase your odds of a good experience by tending to several other details.

Check the characteristics of the course, in particular its ups and downs. Try to remember them and think about your strategy for every mile or 5K stretch.

It's best to prepare everything you can the previous day:

- Choose your running clothes and shoes. Never run in clothes or shoes that you're not used to.
- Cut your toe nails.
- Attach your bib number.
- Prepare extra clothes in case of cold and rain.
- Prepare cap and sunglasses if you're running on a sunny day.

Prepare everything else you want to use during the race, such as fuel belt, gels, and special drinks, GPS watch, MP3 player/smartphone, heart rate monitor, etc. Take everything you really need, but err on the side of minimalism—after twenty miles, everything you carry feels much heavier. Check what will be available at aid stations and don't carry things you'll be able to get on the way.

It often happens that you're so excited the night before the race that you can't sleep well, especially before your first marathon. Then you get worried how you'll be able to run such a long distance having not slept enough, and falling asleep becomes even more difficult. However, if you just lie in bed and let your body rest, there's nothing to worry about. Professor Tanaka and many other experienced marathoners regularly have trouble sleeping the night before a race, and find that once they start running, they feel fine. Getting good sleep every other night in the week before the marathon will increase the chances that tossing and turning the night before won't hurt your energy level on race day.

Day of the Race

Get up early and make sure you have enough time to eat breakfast and get to the start line well in advance. Have your breakfast several hours before running.

Use Band-Aids and Vaseline to prevent chafing in sensitive places, your inner thighs, and nipples.

Apply sunscreen. Even if it's not sunny yet, you're going to spend several hours outside.

Race-Day Meal

Your meal on the day of the race is at least as important as the carbo-loading you do in the days before. It's important to start the big day with a meal that you enjoy and are familiar with. As far as nutrients are concerned, we don't necessarily recommend a meal high in carbohydrates.

If you've carbo-loaded in the previous few days, your glycogen is already accumulated at its maximal possible level and will not get any higher. Our study shows that eating big amounts of carbohydrates again on the day of the race is not only unnecessary, but can also increase your level of blood sugar and insulin, making it difficult for fat to be used as an alternative source of energy.

That's why we recommend a final pre-race meal that's high in fat. It will increase the density of free fatty acid in your blood, help save glycogen, and improve your stamina in the second part of the race. A perfect breakfast before the race, something that is high in fat and protein, could even be a cheeseburger.

Have your breakfast three to four hours before the race. Later, consume only water until the start. Don't consume sugar until just before the race; you can have an energy gel waiting at the start line or just after taking off.

Consider the Conditions

Even with a plan to run at an even pace, you need to be careful about hills, heat, and head wind. Even pace doesn't mean keeping perfectly the same speed; of course you'll slow down when going uphill or into the wind. Wind at your back or going downhill, on the other hand, will help make you feel like you're flying and will very likely boost your speed. Even pacing means keeping the physiological conditions of your body consistent over the course of the race. You can also use a heart rate monitor and control your target number of heart beats per minute to meet this goal.

Hydration and Energy Supplements During the Race

There will probably be aid stations with both water and sport drinks every few miles. That should be enough to stay hydrated— you don't need to carry a heavy bottle with you. Choose sports drinks to prevent dehydration and provide sugar at the same time.

You don't need to swallow huge amounts—half a cup of liquid, consumed in small sips, will be fine. Drinking too much too fast is very likely to result in side stitches or other internal discomfort.

Also, drinking huge amounts, especially of plain water, may result in drastic lowering of the salt density in your blood. This condition, known as hyponatraemia, can have even more serious consequences than dehydration. (See Chapter 9 for more on hyponatraemia.)

If sport drinks aren't available, you can drink water and take an energy gel in the later part of the race. Remember to avoid gels that you've not tried before.

Battle of Body and Mind

Chances are that, once the initial euphoria is over, you'll feel increasingly tired as the miles accumulate, and your body and brain will try to convince you to stop or at least slow down. That's when the marathon becomes so different from other sports. Now it's your head and your heart that need to take the lead, and on them depends your success. We have seen many great runners who theoretically could achieve world-class results, but ultimately didn't because they weren't strong enough mentally. On the flip side, there are thousands upon thousands of runners who don't have great genetics for running, but are superb at blocking out feelings of mental and physical fatigue.

So is there a trick to make you ready for the battle of body and mind that will quite likely happen somewhere along the way?

Being out there alone with the miles ahead and the time passing is tough for all of us. It can become easier with some distractions.

Depending on your goals, you might want to talk to fellow runners. You don't have to tell them your life story, but some simple greetings and a smile can help a lot. Choose carefully who you talk to—earphones are usually a hint that somebody might not be looking for conversation.

If you don't have enough energy to chat, try running next to or behind somebody who seems to be going at a similar pace. You can draw energy from one another, and knowing that you're not the only one suffering means a lot.

It helps to divide the 26.2 miles of a marathon into distances you're familiar with and know you can cover without trouble. For example, it's typical to reach the halfway point and be overwhelmed by the amount of running still in front of you. Try to recall a nice thirteen-mile jog you did that you really enjoyed, perhaps because you felt good or were in a pleasant setting. Tell yourself that all you have to do is replicate that fun run, and you'll be finished the marathon. Use the same technique later; for example, if you have a crisis of spirit at Mile 20, think about a six-mile course you run often to make the remaining distance less daunting. Keep doing that with shorter and shorter familiar distances whenever you hit a rough patch. Divide the distance into smaller parts and run thinking about your next goal—be it the next mile sign or next aid station—instead of the finish line, which always seems too far away.

Music can also help a lot. Some lively beats can give you extra energy, especially in the second part of the race. Check beforehand to make sure your race isn't among those that bans headphones for safety reasons.

Not everyone will be able to finish their first marathon, and even fewer first-timers will be able to run the whole way. But as long as you don't give up after the first attempt and use your failures as lessons, you can still consider your race to be successful.

After the Race

Congratulations! You've done it!

After the emotional moment of crossing the goal line, what you need to do first is to supply water and sugar to your body.

If your legs feel hot or painful, try icing them for five to twenty minutes.

Especially with beginners, muscle damage can be so severe that walking is close to impossible. This is the time to check if you're injured. In a state of post-race euphoria, you might not realize immediately if you're hurt, as compared to simply stiff. Give yourself some time to rest, and then check your body carefully using the M-Test we described in Chapter 7. If there is anything worrying, contact a doctor as soon as possible.

In the meantime, you can always use the very basic RICE method to relieve pain and swelling. RICE stands for rest, ice, compression, and elevation, and this is the sequence in which you should treat your injury.

Even if you're not injured, it's likely that walking and in particular climbing up or down stairs will be difficult in the first days or even weeks after your first marathon. For many of you it will be a pleasant kind of pain, reminding you of your great accomplishment. With each marathon, the post-race pain will be lighter and shorter. For now, enjoy it. It's all part of the experience.

What Next?

We recommend a complete rest for a week after the race. In the case of a course with steep ups and downs, your muscles are damaged and their full recovery might take up to a month. Resume slow jogging when it feels comfortable, but be really careful—not feeling pain or fatigue doesn't always mean that you've fully recovered. For example, research we've done found that testosterone levels in male runners drop significantly the morning after a marathon, and getting back to normal levels takes about a week.

Elite runners usually don't participate in races for the next couple of months. Among amateurs there are many who run races more frequently, but usually some of the races will be just for training or fun. If you ran your race "seriously" you need at the very least two weeks to recover before your next challenge.

A typical recovery plan after the race involves one week of total rest. On the next Sunday you can do a very slow jog for thirty minutes to an hour. The following week you can train similar to how you did in the week before your marathon, except you should skip the midweek long run you might have done pre-race.

What's most important is listening to your body. Relax and do what feels good. Finishing a marathon is a great achievement. Now it's time to reward yourself.

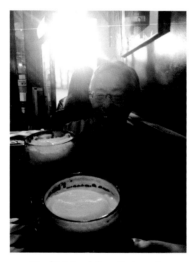

Credit: Magdalena Jackowska

CHAPTER 9

Slow Jogging for Experienced Runners

From the previous chapters you probably see why slow jogging is such a great idea for beginners, and for those whose main goals are health and general fitness. While such runners are a big part of the slow jogging population, this method is also useful for more advanced and ambitious runners. Beginning with Professor Tanaka, there are many competitive runners for whom slow jogging is the foundation of training.

No matter your speed and experience level, we strongly recommend that you learn (or remind yourself of) the importance of listening to your body and avoiding injuries. Between strict training plans and improving your race results, it's a good idea to slow down and analyze your technique; being able to run fast doesn't necessarily mean that you're doing so efficiently.

There's no better way to focus on your technique than running slowly. Forefoot strike, cadence, posture—all the essentials described in this book apply to all runners, no matter their speed. We strongly recommend you spend time to make sure your running technique doesn't do more harm than good, the sooner the better.

Sure, if you're young and fit, poor running technique may not always stop you from getting faster or result in immediate injuries. But that situation isn't going to last forever. Think about and work on it now, not after injury stops you from running for months or years.

Speed is individual and relative. We're not saying to jog at three miles per hour if your usual training speed is six minutes per mile. What we're suggesting is to run at a speed that is slow for you. As long as it's your comfortable and easy pace, it's the slow jogging we're talking about, even if it looks fast to beginners.

Niko Niko and the Marathon

In Chapter 1, we saw how training at *niko niko* pace led to Professor Tanaka running his fastest marathon at the age of fifty. Now let's see how even world-class marathoners benefit from the method.

Frank Shorter

Frank Shorter, the 1972 Olympic Marathon champion and one of the inspirations for the American running boom of the 1970s, was well-known for doing a lot of his training slowly. "My simple, basic theory involves running very easily—at what I call conversational pace—75–90 percent of the time," Shorter wrote in his book *Olympic Gold: A Runner's Life and Times* (1984). Here's a sample of Shorter's training as presented in his book:

Day of the week	AM		PM		Daily distance (mile)
	Training content	Pace (min/mile)	Training content	Pace (min/mile)	
Monday	7 miles	7'00	10 miles	6'30	17
Tuesday	7 miles	6'30~7'00	2 miles warm up 4x 0.75 miles+660yards (intervals)	4'00~4'12	13
Wednesday	7 miles	6'30~7'00	10 miles	6'30	17
Thursday	7 miles	6'30~7'00	0.25 miles x 12 (intervals)	4'00	13
Friday	7 miles	6'30~7'00	10 miles	6'30	17
Saturday	7 miles	6'30~7'00	10 miles or Race	10 miles: 2 mile jog + 7 miles at 5'00 + 1 mile jog	17
Sunday	7 miles	6'30~7'00	20 miles	First half slower than 6'30 or 5'40 Second half 5'00 or under	27

Total weekly distance: 121 miles
Es mated *niko niko* pace: ~5'00

Source: Frank Shorter with Marc Bloom, 1984. Credit: Hiroki Tanaka, Magdalena Jackowska

Calculating from Shorter's best marathon time (2:10:30), we can assume that his target marathon pace is just under five minutes per mile, or about 3:05 per kilometer. As you see, except for interval training on Thursday, his training consisted of running slower than his marathon pace. That easy running represented as much as 97 percent of his total training distance.

Running slowly is vital for elite runners because it allows them to get the miles in while staying fresh for the hard days.

Yuki Kawauchi

This Japanese marathon hero works a full-time job at a high school and has neither official sponsorship nor coach. Usually referred to as "citizen runner," he rose to instant national fame after the 2011 Tokyo Marathon, in which he was the fastest Japanese runner, finishing in 2:08:37.

He's now admired by marathon fans all over the world not only for his fantastic results but also for racing almost every weekend. He is also known for focusing on distance work rather than speed training. On weekdays that are too busy to allow strenuous training, he opts for slow jogging, which, he has said, increases his motivation for weekend training.

In January 2013, Kawauchi came to our institute to determine his *niko niko* pace based on his lactate threshold. At that time it was just below 5:10 per mile. Soon afterwards, having followed Professor Tanaka's advice, he established his new personal record in Beppu Oita (2:08:15, February 2013) and again in Seoul (2:08:14, March 2013).

Let's take a look at his schedule:

Day of the week	AM		PM		Daily distance (mile)
	Training content	Pace (min/mile)	Training content	Pace (min/mile)	
Monday	12 miles	7'25~9'40	-	-	12
Tuesday	12 miles	7'25~9'40	-	-	12
Wednesday	0.6 x 15 (intervals)	4'50~5'00	-	-	9
Thursday	12 miles	7'25~9'40	-	-	12
Friday	12 miles	7'25~9'40	-	-	12
Saturday	13 or 26 miles	13 miles at 5'10 or 26 miles at 6'12	-	-	13 or 26
Sunday	12 miles	7'25~9'40	-	-	12

Total weekly distance: 82-95 miles
Niko niko pace: 5'10

Credit: Hiroaki Tanaka, Magdalena Jackowska

As was Shorter, Kawauchi is an example of a great runner who trains mostly below his target pace, except for one day per week of interval training and races.

Interval training, Tabata, and *Niko Niko* Intervals

Our physical stamina is determined by the functioning of mitochondria in our muscles. That's where the energy source is oxidized, and it is what supplies a lot of the energy needed to run. We already knew about enhancing mitochondria functions through different types of training, but it was only in 1998 that a group headed by Dr. Bruce Spiegelman of Harvard University discovered its enhancement due to switching on the PGC1α gene. At Fukuoka University, we wanted to find out whether PGC1α gene expression increases with exercise at *niko niko* pace. Research on switching it on has been continued since then and led to extremely interesting conclusions. You might have heard of a training method promoted by Dr. Tabata of Doushisha University. His original protocol requires a five-minute warm-up, eight intervals of twenty seconds of maximal intensity exercise followed by ten seconds of rest, and a two-minute cooldown. The subjects in the study were highly trained endurance athletes in peak physical condition. In the study, doing this workout five days a week for six weeks resulted in a 14 percent increase in the participants' aerobic capacity and a 28 percent increase in their anaerobic capacity, thereby providing a significant increase in stamina.

In 2006, Dr. Martin Gibala of McMaster University in Ontario, Canada discovered that maximal exercise like sprinting, repeated five or six times for thirty seconds and alternated with four minutes of rest each time, improved mitochondrial function, and boosted stamina similar to the improvement caused by a more moderate one-hour workout.

We wanted to find out how these results differ from the effects we can expect with safe and easy exercise at *niko niko* pace. Back in 1972, we compared the results of aerobic and anaerobic training with university students. The former consisted of one hour exercise at *niko niko* pace, and the latter of ten repetitions of ten seconds exercise at highest intensity followed by a three-minute break. The results exceeded our expectations: The gains in aerobic capacity were the same with the two types of workouts.

While high-intensity workouts are undoubtedly advantageous for busy people, there are also significant disadvantages. Training at high speed is extremely hard, and carries a high risk of injuries as well as significant stress on your cardiovascular system.

What we can recommend is intervals at your target marathon pace in addition to regular slow jogging. Try five to ten repeats of a half-mile to a kilometer at your marathon pace.

Why Japanese Runners are Good Marathoners

Look at the list of the top 100 runners in the world at 5K, 10K, and the marathon for a given year, and you'll see that the majority of the runners are from East African countries, primarily Kenya and Ethiopia. There are not many Japanese among the 5K and 10K runners, but sometimes as many as twelve of them among marathoners. This seems strange: Theoretically, both long-distance track running and marathons equally depend on runners' aerobic fitness levels.

So how does it happen that Japanese runners excel in marathons but not in races on the track? The answer lies in the training volume—Japanese runners are known for training by running long distances, which helps them to conquer a marathoner's worst nightmare, the "Wall."

Contrary to that of 5Ks and 10Ks, results in a marathon can vary due to glycogen in muscles, which plays a similar role to gasoline for cars. When your body has no more energy available from stored glycogen, you feel sudden weakness and dizziness, and it becomes impossible to maintain your pace.

However, if you run slow enough, your primary source of fuel is fat, and unless you increase your speed you're not going to run out of energy. The higher the speed, the more carbohydrates and less fat you use. That's great news—by choosing a lower speed you can run dozens of miles without hitting the Wall.

There have been some interesting studies on this topic. Danish researchers had people exercise using both legs for one hour, followed by another hour using just one leg. The next day, the subjects exercised for one hour using only the leg not worked unilaterally the day before. They compared the results of training one leg for six days, one hour at a time, with the other leg trained three days, two hours at a time. The results were better for the leg trained three times a week; the reason was a difference in oxidative capacity in muscles and utilization of fat as an alternative source of energy.

Next, Australian researchers divided triathletes into two groups. One trained six times a week and the other three times a week, with the latter group performing a training load equal to what the first group did in two days. Despite doing the same training load, the second group became able to use fat as an alternative source of energy and save glycogen.

As you can see, with long runs at *niko niko* pace, you teach your body to use fat as fuel. That means that in marathons, even if you do run out of glycogen, your body will smoothly switch to fat-fueling like a hybrid car.

Japanese runners who base their training on long distances at relatively low speed are strong marathon runners who are used to maintaining pace even when they run short of gasoline.

Practical Information for Experienced Runners

We have introduced here a bit of theory – let's now look at some scientific tips for marathon running on a slightly more advanced level.

Recovery

The faster and more ambitious runner that you are, the greater the risk of succumbing to a serious injury that will keep you from training like you want. If that happens, some keep training anyway, and ultimately have to stop running for even longer. Some even lose their motivation and enthusiasm, and quit the sport.

Of course, in a perfect world, we wouldn't ever suffer from injuries. That's possible if you listen to your body and think about your technique before and not after you get injured. See Chapter 3 for a refresher on slow jogging basics.

What stops many runners halfway through a promising career is not physical injuries, but psychological burnout. Runners are often ambitious and hard-working individuals. They tend to push themselves to the limits—and sometimes way over the limits. When that happens, running is no longer a pleasure; it becomes a chore you no longer look forward to.

The only way to feel enthusiastic about running again is to change your routine, refresh your running, and remind yourself why you enjoyed it in the first place. Here is where slow jogging comes in handy. The very slow, relaxed pace that will not make you tired even when continued for a long while is a great way to restart your running career. Knowing that exhaustion at the end of the training is not your final goal can really help you rediscover running.

Glycogen Loading

Dr. Per-Olof Åstrand from the Karolinska Institute in Sweden was the first to suggest a specific way for athletes to fill their muscles with glycogen. According to him, one week before a marathon or other long race, you should do a long workout that will use up all your glycogen. For the next three days, eat mostly meals high in protein and fat and low in carbohydrates to keep the level of glycogen in muscles low. Then, three days before the race, eat mostly carbohydrates and avoid intensive exercise. If you follow those steps, Åstrand said, glycogen will accumulate at double the usual amount. This became the classic method of glycogen loading (also known as carbo-loading).

Based on the original studies as well some recent discoveries, we would rather suggest the following method.

Let's suppose that your race is in one week, on a Sunday. On the Sunday before, go for a long run (fifteen miles or more). Do the same on the Wednesday before the race.

Thirty minutes before these two workouts, eat something sugary. That will stimulate insulin secretion, which in turn will inhibit using fat stores to supply energy during exercise. This trick will help you to run out of glycogen faster.

Note: It's possible to achieve the glycogen-depletion results without a long run. For example, run for thirty seconds as fast as you can, rest for five minutes, then do another all-out thirty seconds. Rest for thirty to forty minutes, and repeat the cycle. This method will allow you to get the depletion effects of a twelve-mile jog in less than one mile. Follow it with six miles of slow jogging to get closer to complete depletion.

We recommend not training in the three days before your marathon.

See Chapter 8 for detailed suggestions on carbo-loading.

Warming Up

The world of track and field became interested in the theory of warming up back in the 1940s, when scientists from Northern Europe proved that, for races of 100 to 800 meters, warm-ups can substantially improve performance, by as much as four to eight seconds for an 800-meter race. The runners were able to move fast and supply a lot of energy to their bodies in a short time.

However, marathons are different from track races. Lactate hardly accumulates, and the general pace is quite relaxed. If you run at your average *niko niko* pace, the benefits of warming up are not really relevant.

Let's look at it physiologically. During the days of carbo-loading, you accumulated glycogen in your muscles and at the same time a significant amount of water as well. Warming up, you already start consuming glycogen and eliminate water, and you feel your body getting lighter. That's one of the reasons why many runners feel better standing at the start line having warmed up beforehand.

In the process of glycogen loading you will probably put on a pound or two, so it's only natural that you feel heavy during the first few miles of a marathon. However, if you feel light from the very beginning it only means that you have already depleted your glycogen levels and might not have enough storage to keep the same pace to the finish line.

That's why we very much prefer to consider the first part of the race as the warm-up. This idea was first put forward in the 1960s by the legendary New Zealand coach Arthur Lydiard, who advised walking and trying to relax in the hour before a marathon rather than running at a pace that will drain some of your glycogen stores.

The example of Toshinari Takaoka, who holds the Japanese record in the marathon at 2:06:16, also supports this approach. In 2001, in his first marathon, Takaoka faded in the final miles from 2:07 pace to a finish of 2:09:41. Afterwards, he told Professor Tanaka he had run 5K at marathon pace as part of his warm-up. Professor Tanaka explained why this was a bad idea, and recommended that Takaoka avoid such a warm-up before a marathon. The following year, following that advice, Takaoka set the still-standing Japanese record.

Marathon Pacing Strategy

Generally recommended marathon strategy for more advanced runners is the negative split, which means running the second half of the marathon slightly faster than the first half. This recommendation is based on the physiological facts of glycogen depletion explained above, observation of the most successful elite marathoners, and Professor Tanaka's personal experiences. Try the following for best results:

1. Keep an easy, even pace in the first half of the marathon. Run at 10–11 on the Borg scale, at a pace relaxed enough to hum your favorite songs.
2. From halfway to 30K (18.6 miles), aim for an effort level equating to 11–12 on the Borg scale.
3. From 30K onward, the real racing begins. Between 30K and 35K (21.7 miles), run at a pace equivalent to 12–13 on the Borg scale. From 35K to the finish, aim for 14–16 on the Borg scale, which will more or less be giving it everything you have.

Think of the first eighteen miles as a warm-up and the remaining 8.2 as the actual race!

Dangers of Overhydration

During a marathon, you need to supply your body with both water and sugar. It's of great importance to stay hydrated, but you should also be careful about not drinking too much.

The dangers of doing so became better known after the 2002 Boston Marathon, where a twenty-eight-year-old woman suddenly died during the race. The reason was found to be hyponatremia, which is a low sodium concentration in the blood, and the most common reason for sudden deaths during marathons. This state can be caused by overhydration during the race. Researchers who analyzed data on hypernatremia during that race found that, among 488 examined runners, as many as sixty-six suffered from hypernatremia. The majority of those were runners who finished in 4:00 or slower, and/or were of very slender figure.

During exercise, 70 percent of your energy is used for heat production, so the body temperature rises and, if the weather is hot and humid, you're prone to heatstroke. That's why drinking enough is important. However, the studies suggest that, even if we feel thirsty, drinking at every single water station may result in overhydration and hyponatremia.

So how are we supposed to know the right amount?

In the study at the 2002 Boston Marathon, the subjects were weighed before and after the race. More than 40 percent of the subjects lost more than two pounds, and most of them were among the fastest runners. On the other hand, there were also runners who finished the race eight to ten pounds heavier!

So why do the faster runners lose weight? As you will notice while watching a marathon on TV, unless the race is in really hot weather, the top runners don't usually drink in the first half of the race. Their training has produced adaptations that help them sweat effectively. We can imagine that top runners are quite used to six- to twelve-mile hard runs without drinking. If they were to drink at every water station, they would need to slow each time; doing so and accelerating again every few miles requires extra energy.

Slower runners, in contrast, tend to drink too much water. They probably take a short break at every station and drink plenty.

We suggest checking how much weight you lose when running. Measure it a week before the race, running six to ten miles at a steady pace, without drinking. The weight you lost is almost the equivalent of lost fluids so you should drink a similar or lesser amount to replenish them.

On average, half a cup at every station should be fine. Choose sport drinks if they're available to supply sugar as well. If they're not available, you might want to consume an energy gel around Mile 20, but be careful not to eat those you're not used to.

CHAPTER 10

Slow Jogging Success Stories

L et's now hear from runners of different ages, nationalities, and abilities, all of whom have one thing in common—they've accomplished their varying achievements thanks to slow jogging. We've grouped individual success stories by broad categories such as improved health and weight loss.

Feeling Better

I cannot imagine a more anti-running person than myself. At least that was the case until several months ago, but now that has changed, and I do several miles of slow jogging every week.

I have heard many times that I'm "pretending to run" or "maybe do not have energy today," but now I think it's almost part of the fun. "Slow" is my way to think not just about running, but about an active and healthy life in general.

I don't have a lot of time in my everyday life; that's why slow jogging works perfectly for me. I always jog when walking my dog and going shopping nearby. My mother recently started to slow jog in the house while vacuuming! My favorite method is slow jogging while chatting with my friends.

We are never going to have enough time to do everything we want. I learned to use the time between other activities for slow jogging!

(Woman, forties)

***

My daughter was the one who started promoting slow jogging outside of Japan, so I couldn't possibly not become interested in it. And even before she did, she was experimenting on me.

I had never run or jogged before; I always considered it to be a sport for those younger and fitter. I am in my sixties and used to lose my breath climbing the stairs. But slow jogging is a different story! I was able to do it, and after several days I got used to it and felt comfortable. Of course at the beginning I was walking quite a bit, but soon enough I could jog my regular lap in the nearby forest without stopping. Now I slow jog every day if I have enough time and the weather is good; if not, a couple of times a week.

I feel really good knowing that I'm doing something for my body and my fitness. And after my first month of slow jogging, I wasn't getting out of breath on the stairs that easily! Highly recommended!

(Woman, sixties)

***

Today was my first time to take part in a slow jogging event. I'm in my fifties and I had never tried slow jogging before, but I knew I wanted to do it. I want to feel young again, just like Professor Tanaka does. I'm going to tell all my friends about this interesting and accessible sport that we can even do at home.

I'm impressed by the results we can achieve with slow jogging, especially those related to the memory and brain fitness.

(Five months after the first meeting, H. contacted us again. She keeps slow jogging and enjoys it a lot!)
(Woman, fifties)

Health Improvement and Weight Loss

My experience with slow jogging started three years ago. I started walking for exercise twenty years ago and tried slow jogging after watching *Tameshite Gatten*, a well-known educational program on Japanese television. The results were more than clear. My health improved in many aspects, including my level of triglycerides, type of fats found in blood, (decreased from 500–600 to 160–200 mg/dL) and blood sugar level (from 100–110 to 80–95 mg/dL).

At first I used to run at three to four miles per hour, but after some time it changed to five to six miles per hour. I can still talk and I am never short of breath!
(Man, sixties)

***

I'm in my forties. Slow jogging not only helped me to overcome depression but also made me healthier in my body and mind.

These are the results I experienced:

- Recovery from depression and no relapses
- Less feelings of sadness and anger
- Feeling more active and energetic
- Less pain and stiffness in my neck, shoulders, back, and legs
- My stomach is flatter and firmer
- My skin looks better

I believe it's a great cure-all!
(Woman, forties)

***

I'm not that young anymore, and two years ago I started to exercise every morning in the park, in order to improve my health.

At first I was doing a mixture of tai-chi and other types of Eastern and Western exercise. By chance I heard about slow jogging and added ten minutes to my everyday routine, but at first I didn't experience any significant health benefits.

A year later I tried to jog more. I usually started with some warm-up exercise, did thirty minutes of slow jogging and stretched afterwards. Now I jog every day, even when it's raining.

I feel great and my check-up results have never been better. These are the changes in the last few months:

- Uric acid: from 9.5 to 6.8 mg/dL
- Total cholesterol: from 256 to 167 mg/dL
- High blood pressure that I suffered from for more than ten years got gradually lower, and I was able to stop taking medication for it. My blood pressure is stable now, with systolic 100–120 and diastolic 55–70 mm Hg.
(Man, eighties)

***

I have always disliked sports, and running in particular. I started with slow jogging after work, two to three times a week. To be honest, at the beginning I was having quite a hard time.

Gradually jogging while listening to music became easier and sometimes even enjoyable. The pounds I was losing became my great motivation! Now I am used to it and can keep jogging even without the thirty-second walk I used to take every minute.

I also kept in mind all the suggestions about meals and calories and lost four-and-a-half pounds per month on average. My weight at the beginning was 174, and now it's 161. I don't remember the last time I needed to buy new clothes in a smaller size!

(Man, twenties)

***

Ten years ago, at sixty-five, I retired and soon afterwards had a health check at a local hospital. I was told I was at risk of chronic diseases and metabolic syndrome and was told to lose weight.

Five years ago, at seventy, I participated in a slow jogging event, but wasn't really able to stick to the exercise routine and soon went back to my old habits and weight.

This year I decided to try it again and participated in a three-day slow jogging and diet retreat. It was a very hard schedule but I understood the principles of jogging at *niko niko* pace, without pushing myself. During the retreat I already lost a pound.

After the retreat, I kept with daily slow jogging. I believe that consistency is the key, and went jogging even on rainy or windy days. This time it was easier, because I bought slow jogging shoes designed by Professor Tanaka, and they made it much simpler to land on the forefoot.

My everyday routine at first was to slow jog before breakfast or lunch for sixty minutes and do slow step exercise before dinner. I was advised to aim at 20,000 steps a day so I changed my plan to sixty minutes slow jogging before breakfast and another sixty minutes before lunch or dinner.

Last fall I ran in my first 5K (3.1-mile) race. Until then I would usually alternate jogging and walking, so it was my first experience of jogging continuously. I finished pretty tired after forty minutes.

I wanted to try running continuously so I started having fewer walking periods in my training—first, every seven minutes, later every fifteen minutes until I was able to run thirty minutes without having to stop.

Two months after I started, I had lost eleven-and-a-half pounds. After four months, I'd lost twenty-one pounds.

I think the most difficult part for me was to be cautious about calories. I would exercise before breakfast but then eat too much afterwards. Now my main purpose is just to stay healthy and enjoy the balance of nice food in reasonable quantities and slow jogging.

(Man, seventies)

***

First Marathons and Half Marathons

Going to the train station, from the station to the office, lunch break, evening after work, weekends—for me, every moment is a good time for slow jogging!

When I started, that wasn't the case. Every minute of jogging felt like eternity, people were walking faster than I jogged, and I was embarrassed. But at the end of my first week I started to feel different. I was refreshed and had more energy. I used to weigh 166 pounds; now it's 159, and my friends say I look slimmer. I notice it as well.

A few months after starting slow jogging, I entered my first half marathon—and finished it! I'm thinking of a full marathon in the near future.

I started slow jogging only a few years ago, but it's already one of the main pleasures in my life and big part of everyday life.

(Woman, forties)

***

At fifty, I was diagnosed with light hypertension, diabetes, and a fatty liver, and advised to exercise. I went to Professor Tanaka's lecture and decided to give running a try. I started with a slow jog of around three miles once a week.

When I was fifty-six, I attended an event for people who might want to run the Honolulu Marathon, which is run in December. That August, I decided to run twice a week, gradually extending the distance. Starting that November, I trained three times a week. My monthly distance was fifty miles in August, sixty miles in September, sixty-eight miles in October, and seventy-five miles in November.

During this time my weight dropped from 149 to 129 pounds. The results of my next medical check were within the norm for all of my previous health problems.

One month before the race, I caught a bad cold and wasn't able to train as I wanted to. I was anxious, but tried to focus on what I have learned about preparation, nutrition and even pacing. I completed my first marathon in 4:34, feeling very happy.

(Man, fifties)

**

I decided to start running when I was on a trip to India. I was twenty-seven at the time. Faced with the harsh reality of life and death in India, I got to thinking seriously about what it means to be fully alive. One of the things I always wanted to do was run a marathon, so after returning from India, I planned to run the Honolulu Marathon and started training at a sports club.

My first marathon took 5:24. Later I completed ultramarathons of 100 kilometers (sixty-two miles) and 150 miles. I completed all the races I was dreaming about and wanted to run faster. I enrolled in workshops led by Professor Tanaka. Five months later, I ran my first sub-4:00 marathon, improving my previous best by almost an hour. After another three months, I ran 3:39. My next goal is to break 3:30.

(Woman, thirties)

**

Around ten years ago I broke my leg. I put on weight and for a long time couldn't get rid of the pain. I started using a cane whenever going outside.

At sixty-three I heard about step exercise and slow jogging for the first time and decided to try them. In the first couple of months I did only the step exercise, but as my condition improved I started slow jogging as well. At that time I finally started walking without my cane again. During that time I lost eighteen pounds.

Jogging was getting not only easier but also more fun, and the following year I joined the classes that were preparing for the Honolulu Marathon with the slow jogging method. Six months later I flew to Honolulu and completed the marathon.

Becoming able to run after years of walking with a cane gave me a lot of confidence. Even more than finishing a marathon, that's the most important change I experienced since I started slow jogging.

(Woman, sixties)

Stunning Running Performances

I ran track and cross country in high school and did triathlons in college. I didn't run or exercise much in my thirties but started running again when I turned forty. I pushed myself just about every time I trained. My hard training made me stronger, faster, leaner, and stronger, but often left me exhausted.

Early one morning, I ran with a group of runners who jogged more than two minutes per mile slower than my normal pace. I quickly became impatient and wanted to go faster, but I stayed with them.

Halfway through, I realized how happy everyone was, and what great conversations they were having. It's hard to smile or talk about something fun when you're running above lactate threshold with three other sweaty guys. But when you slow down, you can have a quality conversation or, if you're alone, meditate about something important in your life. A good slow jog with friends is a great way to start the day.

I still do hard runs, but now only two times a week. I go more slowly on my other training runs, whether I'm alone or with my slow jogging buddies. Going slow leaves me refreshed rather than exhausted, lets me push myself harder when I do run fast, and isn't as hard on my body so I can continue my favorite pastime well into old age (I hope).

If you think slow jogging is for the weak-willed or lackadaisical, take the example of one of my slow jogging buddies. He's over fifty and always keeps his pace at ten minutes per mile or slower, but since he doesn't zap his muscles and joints with hard running, he's able to run as much as he wants. In fact, he's run over 500 miles in a month, yet he still runs sub-3:30 marathons.

(Man, forties)

***

During my university days I competed professionally in kendo, a martial arts-inspired sport involving bamboo poles. I continued practicing after graduating but later on, busy with my work at a bank, I became sedentary and put on nine pounds.

One day out of nowhere I received an invitation to run a half marathon for charity. It was a point-to-point course starting on a mountain and descending towards the seashore. Being heavy, I almost rolled down towards the finish line and completed the course in 1:50.

That's when I met Professor Tanaka. He told me about his slow jogging theory, and I decided to give it a try.

My first marathon was in 1994. Before the race I ran on average fifty-five miles a month, at *niko niko* pace or below. We measured my lactate threshold, and based on the results I was given a pre-dicted time of 3:30. You can imagine how unreal it felt!

To my great surprise I finished in 3:34, and got seriously addicted to running. I gradually started running longer distances and started losing weight as well. The following year, fourteen pounds lighter, I broke 3:00.

I kept training at *niko niko* pace and was running around 120 miles per month. I finished my next marathon in 2:52, and I know I can get even faster!

(Man, forties)

***

I always enjoyed playing tennis, and that might be why I com-pleted my first marathon in 3:55 after training for just a couple of months.

I was not fat at all, but Professor Tanaka told me that 101 to 103 pounds would be my optimal running weight. Three months later, at a weight of 108, I ran 2:59.

With practically every race I was getting faster. In the fall of that year, I ran 2:43, an almost unbelievable time for an amateur woman, or so I was told. I weighed 101 pounds at that time and finished in twenty-first place. I was forty years old, and had been running for only two years.

Two years after that, I got even faster, running 2:40. I was very happy, and couldn't have accomplished that without studying the sport and having great advisors, including Professor Tanaka.

As for my training method, I usually never ran faster than my slow jogging pace, which is between 9:00 and 10:00 per mile.

Now I am an exchange student in Honolulu and have been finishing near the top of my age group in the Honolulu Marathon for a couple of years in a row!

(Woman, forties)

***

I have been running all my life. I'm a woman, and my fastest marathon is 2:38.

In high school I started experimenting with longer distances, and I ran my first marathon at age twenty-two. Back then I was a student at Fukuoka University, and my coach was Professor Tanaka.

Slow jogging has always been and will be the base of my training. It's by far the best way to learn the running technique and rhythm without risking overtraining. Forefoot landing, correct posture and rhythm should be learned as early as possible; speed is something you can always work on later.

I ran my fastest marathon as a university student, but now, in my thirties, I still run around 2:40. My technique hasn't changed, and is the same whether I jog or race.

During a slow jogging event, I met my future husband. A few years later we became the Guinness World Record holders for the fastest marathon run by a married couple, with the aggregate time of 5:28:23 in the 2014 Tokyo Marathon.

Just give slow jogging a try. You never know what's in store for you!

(Woman, thirties)

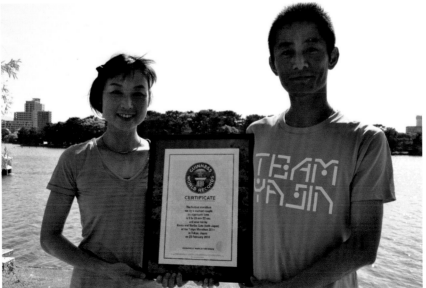

Credit: Noriko Satou

CHAPTER 11
Slow Jogging FAQs

n this chapter, we provide detailed answers to the most common questions people have about slow jogging.

Q: I plan to do slow jogging but I end up running too fast. Is there any trick to keep running at the correct pace?

A: Keeping the proper, consistent pace is extremely important. It's very helpful to choose a running location with distance indicators or run laps measuring the time, especially at the beginning, when you are having difficulties keeping the same pace.

There are also various smartphone apps that let you track your pace per mile and store your running data. These are not only a great help for beginners during runs but also help you to keep track of your fitness and progress.

Another option is running on a treadmill. It may not be particularly exciting, but as far as keeping a steady pace is concerned, the treadmill does the job for you. You can always switch back to running outside when you feel your body remembers the pace.

Q: Is it enough to just jog? Shouldn't I be doing some kind of muscle or strength training as well?

A: The biggest muscles in the human body are the quadriceps, back muscles, hips and waist area, and inner abdominal muscles. They are all working when slow jogging at a high enough rate to prevent muscle degradation.

Whether you should supplement slow jogging with weight-lifting depends on your fitness goals. If you are dreaming of a bodybuilder-like physique, slow jogging itself is not going to get you there. If your purpose is weight loss, general fitness or/and becoming a faster runner, then slow jogging will provide all the training you need.

Of course, muscle training in moderation will not harm! It's not essential, but as is the case with any kind of exercise, is worth trying.

However, if you're a runner and want to improve your speed, be careful with upper-body strength training. Developing a very muscular upper body means you will have to carry more weight, and could slow you down.

Q: My goal is a sub-3:00 marathon. What kind of training do you recommend? How long will it take?

A: Many non-professional runners dream of a sub-3:00 marathon. It requires running at an average speed close to nine miles per hour, so it's highly unlikely for amateurs to be able to achieve it without enough preparation. But the training method is not very different from what we recommend for slower runners—the base is your current *niko niko* pace. Of course, the time you will need to achieve your goal varies greatly, depending on your initial fitness.

Let's assume that you're an experienced runner who currently runs a marathon in 3:15 and wants to break 3:00. The main elements you will have to work on are your aerobic capacity, efficient use of fat as alternative source of energy, light body weight, and improvement of running skills.

Of those, the easiest element to work on is usually attaining an optimal racing weight.

Let's suppose that you weigh 170 pounds now. Dropping fifteen pounds will make a sub-3:00 marathon possible. This can be accomplished in four to six weeks.

First, slightly reduce your everyday caloric intake, preferably by 300–400 calories; for example, reduce 150–200 calories at breakfast and lunch. Eat more proteins than usual, but try to cut out carbohydrates and fats. As far as the evening meal is concerned, you don't need to make any particular changes or cuts.

Your recommended daily running distance during that time will be seven to ten miles, and the training basis will be slow jogging. In addition to that, twice a week you can try the following interval training: Five to eight repeats of one mile each, with a half-mile recovery jog between at a very easy pace. Start at 7:20 per mile for the first session, and run the repeats twenty seconds per mile faster every two weeks.

When you don't have time for your regular training, use the spare time throughout the day to alternate one minute of slow jogging with thirty seconds of walking. Jog and walk on the way to and from work, do two or three sets every half hour at work (going to the toilet, getting a coffee, etc.), at lunchtime and so on. One set of mixed slow jogging and walking covers about 130 yards. This jogging-in-the-meantime trick can give you as much as ninety sets accumulated during the day, which is almost seven miles covered.

If you follow the plan above, you can expect to lose weight as well as teach your body to be more efficient at using fat as a fuel source. At that point, you will be ready to give sub-3:00 a go. Good luck!

Q: Is it really possible to prepare for a sub-3:00 marathon training with just slow jogging/at *niko niko* pace?

A: Yes. *Niko niko* pace intensity is sufficient to improve your maximal oxygen uptake and fat metabolism. At the same time, *niko niko* pace (or even slower) is optimal for running long distances and losing weight, which will get you closer to your time goal.

Niko niko pace is also comfortable enough for you to be able to concentrate on your technique and running skills; a faster pace will make doing so close to impossible.

There are elite runners who train mostly at their *niko niko* pace. See the last section of Chapter 10 for examples.

Q: You talk about interval training, which in my mind constitutes pretty hard and advanced training. What does interval training mean in the context of *niko niko* pace and slow jogging?

A: Intervals as such do not necessarily mean running at certain speeds, high or low. Instead, it's a way to divide the training into the relatively faster periods interspersed with slower recovery periods that allow your body to rest after the harder part.

Your pace, distance, and the number of repetitions in each part are all flexible and depend on your fitness goals.

The intervals for complete beginners we recommend are alternating one minute of slow jogging with thirty seconds of walking. You can do these almost any place at any time; you probably won't sweat. But don't underestimate their effectiveness!

Their simplicity makes it easy to accumulate many sets throughout the day, and they can be a powerful tool in losing weight and improving fitness.

For more advanced runners, we recommend half-mile intervals at their *niko niko* pace alternated with very slow jogs for a similar distance, repeated 7–10 times.

Q: I'm pretty heavy right now. Isn't it better to lose some weight first and then start running?

A: That's one way to do it. Studies have found an average weight loss of about two pounds per month from dieting. Those who started running after three months of dieting at this level of weight loss say they feel lighter and that running is easier.

Having said that, if your primary purpose is weight loss, the most effective way is exercise and diet combined. It allows an average loss of two pounds in ten days. We recommend small breakfasts and lunches (about 300 calories each) and dinner of your choice. That, combined with three miles of slow jogging every day, makes a loss of one pound in five days possible.

Q: I'm pregnant. Is it safe for me to jog?

A: Yes. As long as slow jogging feels comfortable, there's no reason to avoid it during pregnancy. It will help to prevent excessive weight gain and also strengthen your core muscles, which are crucial during child birth.

Q: What if I'm too old for running?

A: There's no such thing as being too old for running. Quite the contrary: the older you are, the more important it is that you exercise.

Many of us exercise less as we grow older. But our bodies grow older because we exercise less and less! We have seen many people who started jogging at age sixty, seventy, or eighty after decades of a sedentary lifestyle. Some of them have even run marathons by now.

Q: I tried slow jogging and injured my knee. How should I cope with it, and is there a way to prevent getting hurt in the future?

A: A frequent cause of knee injuries is heel striking. If that's the case, switching to forefoot/midfoot strike is the best solution and treatment at the same time. Remember to keep your steps short and your body straight when landing; imagine a pole from the top of your head, one that goes through your waist and hips to the balls of your feet. Try contracting the front and back part of your thigh muscles at the same time.

In the case of severe injuries or illnesses, it's always a good idea to ask your doctor, but the general rule for slow jogging is: As long as you can walk (with no pain nor discomfort) you can also try slow jogging. Start at a very low speed and walk for thirty seconds after every minute of jogging. It's a very light exercise that can even help you with rehabilitation, but if at any point you feel pain—don't push it.

If the pain is really bad, stop running until it feels better. In the meantime, do step exercise with a rail for support, cycling, or swimming instead.

Q: Is there any difference between running outside and running on the treadmill?

A: While the treadmill doesn't simulate your natural stride perfectly, it's close enough to provide an efficient training alternative.

That means that the main difference between running outside and on the treadmill is your preference. Treadmills make it easy to keep a steady pace and do your intervals at target speeds. If you are a beginner and have trouble keeping a slow, steady pace, they can be quite useful.

If you are a more advanced runner, try to set your marathon pace in the pace settings, run for a couple of minutes, than change the pace to one mile per hour lower for thirty seconds to one minute, then repeat the cycle.

Another option worth trying on the treadmill is the incline. It gives you a chance to practice more challenging settings as well as providing a great lower-body workout. Unless you can't stand the idea of indoor running hamster-style, treadmills give you an opportunity to play with the pace and incline in a way that would be difficult when jogging outside.

Basically, it's up to you. Choose one or the other or do both, depending on your training plan on a given day, the weather, etc.

Q: What's the best surface to run on? Asphalt? Track? Trails?

A: As long as you are landing correctly on the forefoot, it doesn't really make a big difference. The impact force and stress on the joints are relatively small, even if you're running on asphalt. However, running on grass or sand stimulates the biggest number of running muscles, so can be more beneficial physiologically.

And while technically we don't have anything against running on asphalt or concrete, it's quite likely you will enjoy it more if you find a dirt path surrounded by the trees or along the beach.

Q: My area gets really cold in winter. What should I wear when running outside in winter?

A: If the temperature is lower than 40 degrees Fahrenheit, you might want to wear some extra protection. The clothes should be comfortable to move in, so choose apparel that offers enough warmth but are not too bulky. Take your gloves with you and use them when necessary.

As soon as you start running, 70 percent of the energy produced will escape as heat, so you should start feeling nice and warm soon.

Q: What about when it's raining hard or other bad weather situations?

A: Some of us don't mind or even enjoy running in the rain, especially in the warmer months. Still, for many people bad weather conditions can be a reason (or good excuse) to give up training.

Some areas will give you a hard time in the winter, whereas in others the heat and humidity make jogging in the summer difficult and sometimes dangerous.

So should you just take a break, or maybe use a treadmill at the gym or at home? For those willing to experiment, we have another idea: Try jogging across the room without stepping on a treadmill! Crazy as it may sound, it's doable and even has some advantages over regular jogging.

Yoichi Hatamoto, PhD, of our fitness institute proved that turns, necessary for running back and forth, significantly increase energy expenditure and help shape up your body. Decreasing speed before a turn, turning the body and regaining the original speed mean that a shuttle jog at two-and-a-half miles per hour over a distance of ten feet and with twenty turns per minute is physiologically equivalent to running at three-to-four miles per hour in a straight line or on the treadmill.

Continuing it for thirty minutes can be hard for some, but a couple of minutes several times a day is doable. Here again, try slow jogging in intervals (one minute of jogging and thirty seconds of walking) if you're not confident.

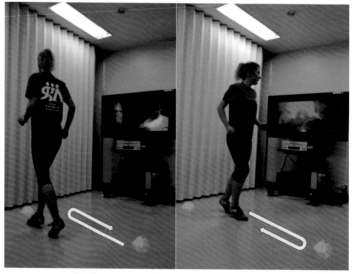

Credit: Kazumi Takeo, Magdalena Jackowska

Give it a try now: Measure ten feet on the floor and have a go, barefoot, or maybe even while watching TV!

Q: I can't afford to buy new shoes for slow jogging right now. I have some regular thick-soled sneakers, hiking shoes, and Converse trainers. Would any of these work?

A: You should be fine with your Converse trainers. If you are not sure, try the shoes you have to see which pair feels most similar to being barefoot. Thin and flexible soles will definitely be beneficial. If you have a safe path nearby, try running with no shoes at all—there's no better way to feel and understand how your body works when running. Just be careful about where you step.

Q: I would like to use a heart rate monitor. Which one should I choose, and how can I use it to find out my optimal slow jogging pace?

A: Unless it's a really cheap one, those devices don't really differ that much, so any brand will do.

Try running at an effort level of 10–12 on the Borg scale we introduced in Chapter 2. Check your heart rate after three to four minutes. It should be around 138 - (your age divided by two). If it's lower, try running again a little bit faster and check your heart rate after another three to four minutes.

If you use this formula, but the exercise intensity feels like 13 or more on the Borg scale, try to recalculate using 128 - (your age divided by two).

On the contrary, if the original formula feels too easy (9 or less on the scale) change it to 148 - (your age divided by two).

If you continue training, the heart rate at a given speed will get lower, so a heart rate monitor can be useful to see your progress.

Once a month get on a treadmill and run for four minutes at a pace that you feel is your *niko niko* pace. Then make it a half-mile per hour faster, run another four minutes, and make it a half-mile per hour faster again. Check your heart rate three times, just before or just after finishing the four minutes at every speed, and make notes.

Compare your results with previous months. A lower heart rate for the same speed shows that your fitness has improved and your training has been effective.

Also, if you lose weight, that alone is enough to lower your heart rate for the same speed.

Q: I would like to run a race. Should I run a marathon or half marathon? Do you recommend starting with a 10K?

A: The typical approach is to start with a 5K (3.1 miles) or 10K (6.2 miles) and proceed to a half marathon and marathon later on.

However, we don't all have time to participate in frequent races, and there aren't always a lot of races available locally. If you're prepared and feel ready, it's okay to run a marathon as your first race. Just make sure that you have covered distances like 10K or half marathon as part of your training.

Q: Is there something I should pay attention to in my everyday diet as a runner? How many calories, and how many carbohydrates, do you recommend**?**

A: If you're running three miles a day or more, you can eat according to your appetite and common sense. Try to keep carbohydrates to 30 percent of your total caloric intake. Also try to eat 0.5–1 gram of protein per one pound of your body weight, especially fish and soy/beans, daily. Eat as many vegetables as you want. For dessert, choose fruit-based ones.

However, if your main reason to start jogging is weight loss, you'll need to plan your menu more carefully. See Chapter 6 for more details.

Q: I want to try the diet style you recommend, but for many years I have been eating a big breakfast and small dinner, so switching to the way you recommend will be very difficult and unrealistic for me. Can I change the order of the meals?

A: Yes. Our usual recommendation of small breakfasts and lunches and big evening meals is designed to fit the busy lifestyle of those who don't have enough time for proper breakfasts and lunches. For them it's relatively easy to have less food during the day, but they want to enjoy a nice, slow meal after a long day at work.

However, what really counts is the total calories you consume in a day, so you're welcome to turn the plan around and enjoy your hearty breakfasts. You can also have smaller portions more times during the day, as long as you stick to the calorie balance and slow jogging schedule.

Q: What should I do about morning and noon meals when traveling or away on business?

A: Try choosing products high in protein and low in carbohydrates, such as plain yogurt, fruits, vegetables, or protein shakes and bars. If you're following our diet plan, make sure you don't exceed the usual number of calories for breakfast (300 calories). If you do, adjust your meals later on during the day.

Q: My work requires attending many events or business dinners. It's nearly impossible to keep track of the number of calories I consume on those days.

A: We all have situations when it's difficult to precisely estimate the number of calories we eat. It became much easier with smartphone apps like MyFitnessPal, but checking the exact calories of a steak during an official business dinner is not always an option.

Try to follow several basic rules and you will be fine. Choose a variety of side dishes instead of standard-size portions, preferably based on fish, meat, eggs, or tofu. Use lemon or non-oil dressing for your salad. Avoid carbs and fried dishes. Have as many green vegetables as you wish.

Q: I tried slow jogging for the first time and the next day I had sharp pain in my calves. Is this normal?

A: Running on the midfoot activates different muscles than heel striking, so if you have been a heel striker so far, a sudden change of technique is likely to result in muscle pain. Allow yourself some transition time and gradually increase the frequency and distance of midfoot running.

Also make sure you understand where the forefoot/midfoot is. We have seen many runners who were so focused on kicking the heel striking habit that they ended up running on their toes, which is extremely dangerous and has nothing to do with correct running form.

Try a series of jumps and jog barefoot and backwards until you're sure you feel what part of your feet you should be landing on. If possible, use barefoot-style shoes, which will help you to get the midfoot habit before you know it.

Q: I heard that after running I should have a nutritious meal. Are there any particular kinds of food you recommend eating after running?

A: Actually, the nutritional priority after exercise is to rehydrate, with water or a sports drink. As for meals, make sure that you supply your body with carbohydrates to help restore glycogen as well as protein to recover and rebuild muscle tissue. Choose simple products such as rice, bread, or pasta to refuel carbohydrates and low-fat meat or fish, prepared with no extra fat, for protein.

Remember to be realistic about the quantity. All of the above is important after a long running session, but not necessary after a short walk and jog with your dog.

Q: Is it a good idea to go slow jogging with my dog?

A: Sure. Jogging solo can be lonely, and your jogging buddies might not always have time for you. Your perfect companion might be the one you live with—your dog, who will never refuse a jog or complain that it's too early, cold, rainy, etc. He might even be the one convincing you to go.

Remember that, just like you, your dog needs to get used to exercise, so take it slow. Always have his leash and water for both of you. Don't go jogging when it's too hot, and contact your vet if there is anything worrisome.

If you both get into it, check out enjoyable sports for both of you such as Cani-cross or dog trekking.

Q: I've tried to count my steps but I only get thirty or thirty-five in fifteen seconds. Is it really necessary to get to forty-five or more? What's the purpose?

A: It's easy to increase your step frequency (also known as cadence) to forty-five or more in fifteen seconds (or 180 per minute) if you take really small steps. That, in turn, will make a forefoot landing more natural. Also, if you're into racing, a higher cadence allows you a more efficient running technique that will help you save energy for the later miles of a race.

Q: I've been told that it's best to have a day off after running to recover. Does this principle apply to slow jogging?

A: Not really. If your slow jogging technique is correct and you don't exceed your *niko niko* pace, you're not risking muscular damage and fatigue that would require a long recovery time. (You can consider a rest day if you feel particularly tired after a long jog.)

It's true, however, that a recovery period is essential after high-intensity training. Not only does it give you a chance to rest, but also puts your body in a state of super-compensation, during which your fitness surpasses its initial level.

Q: Is stretching important in the case of slow jogging?

A: It never hurts to warm up a bit before exercise. Slow jogging, however, is a very gentle form of exercise, so it's enough to stretch the main muscles in your legs, start walking, and proceed to jogging. If you're on a more intense training session, slow jogging itself is a great warm-up.

Q: How can I make running seem less boring?

A: While the process of jogging itself is indeed repetitive, there are many ways to make the experience more exciting. Run different courses or at a different time of day. When you have more time, run on easy trails and enjoy the beautiful views. If you are in a new place, jogging is a great way to get to know the area.

Indoors, when you can watch TV while running on a treadmill, the possibilities are endless.

If none of the above sounds appealing, you can always take a pragmatic approach of running to or from work.

For many people, jogging is an irreplaceable time to be alone with their thoughts and to run away from everyday problems. Unlike classes at a gym, it's a great chance to refresh without having to focus on complicated choreography.

Otherwise, listening to music is probably the most common way to make the experience less monotonous and give you some extra stimulus on the way. Getting a running buddy is also great;

when absorbed in conversation, you'll not even notice the time passing. Chatting when slow jogging also shows whether your pace is relaxed enough.

If nothing of the above seems to help, there's no need to push yourself to run daily. Try step exercise, cycling, or swimming every other day.

Once jogging becomes your habit, the initial "boredom" is likely to turn into a chance to observe the world around you that you have been missing so far. You will be there to see the world waking up or going to sleep and to witness the changes in seasons.

CHAPTER 12

Final Thoughts for a Lifetime of Successful Slow Jogging

By now, you know all the theory you need to enjoy the slow jogging experience. Before you embark on your journey, here are some final tips.

- Set specific goals and rewards for achieving them. If your main target is weight loss, decide on a number of pounds you first want to lose, and then set a realistic, but specific amount of time in which to do so.
- Set challenging but attainable goals. Don't aim too high too soon. It's easier to succeed starting with small steps, and set a more ambitious goal next time.
- Make slow jogging an activity that you look forward to rather than a dreaded routine. Choose a morning jog to get a boost of energy that lasts all day. Or go for a calming jog before bed to relax and make the stress of the day go away. If occasionally you're really not in the mood to run, don't push yourself. You'll

soon be surprised how your body misses activity and be even happier to go jogging the following day.

- The world isn't going to end if you don't exercise or forget about your diet for one day. Forgive yourself for occasional lapses. Don't make it an excuse, but remember that what you want to achieve are lifelong goals, so one less successful day won't undo the good job you've been doing for weeks and will keep working on.

- Make it easy to go for a jog without wasting a lot of time getting ready. Prepare your running shoes and clothing the night before if your jog is in the morning, or carry these items with you whenever you have a while to spare. If you're just jogging for ten minutes between daily activities, you don't even need that. Just make sure you have a bottle of water at hand.

- Find what approach to jogging best suits you. Decide whether you want to jog alone or with a buddy, listen to music if you want, jog in the morning, evening, or during the day, use fancy equipment and clothes, or just your old sweatpants. There's no right or wrong here as long as you enjoy it and stick with it.

- Use an activity tracking app or keep a training log. It'll be great motivation to see how far you've come over time. Track changes in your body weight as well. This will fluctuate on a day-to-day basis so look for the long-term trend.

- Always look at the big picture. Yes, it would be great to get a bikini-ready body in a couple of days and miraculously be able to keep it forever, but that's not likely to happen. You're probably going to have ups and downs, feel motivated or not, sometimes lose weight, and sometimes put it back on. Don't be too hard on yourself and give up after small failures. We're talking about a lifelong purpose here, so sticking to it long-term is what counts most.

- Don't get easily discouraged and don't worry about what others think. We can tell you straight away that when you slow jog, surprised walkers may overtake you and hard-core runners may laugh. What counts is that you're out there realizing your goals. You're much more likely to achieve them jogging at an ultra-slow speed than sitting on your couch.

- Try to find a local jogging group. Even if on most days you'll be jogging on your own, it gives you extra structure and motivation to join a group once every week or two.

- If you have no trouble walking, you're fit enough to do slow jogging. If your current weight, age, or condition raises concerns about starting an exercise routine, consult your physician or exercise physiologist. Make sure to explain that you're planning to do slow jogging, which is no more stressful to your heart and joints than going for a walk.

- Focus on overall activity. For faster health and weight-loss results, don't only add the jogging routine to your life, but think about your existing habits. Jog, walk, or cycle instead of driving everywhere. Take the stairs instead of the elevator. Remember that all your household tasks like cleaning or gardening add greatly to your total daily energy expenditure. Take a break at the office every hour or two to stand up from your desk and take a one-minute slow jog, two or three times a day if that is possible. Consider getting a stand-up desk.

- What counts is now. The past is in the past. If you haven't been eating healthfully and exercising for quite a while and feel regret and guilt about your condition and appearance, try to forget it. What you need to work on is present condition. No matter how bad your fitness level is and how many extra pounds you have to lose, now is when things will start to change. You just need to really want it, plan it, and commit to it.

- Sign up for a race well in advance. It can be just a 5K, but knowing that it's on your calendar and you have already paid for it can motivate more than you'd think.

- Commit financially. Investing in running gear, a gym membership, or a supply of healthy snacks can be helpful when the motivation just doesn't seem to be there.
- Learn to predict the obstacles that you'll constantly face and work through them. If you know that in the evening you're likely to feel too tired to go for a jog, plan it for the morning instead. If you know that you have dinner plans that will likely sabotage your diet, adjust your total daily calories accordingly or/and go for a longer jog.
- It's never too late. The sooner you start, the better. How about now?

Professor Tanaka has traveled a lot in America and Europe, and always enjoys the beautiful views and parks that these locales have to offer. He finds them perfect for a slow, relaxing jog. What always surprises him is that the runners he meets abroad don't seem to enjoy the environment or the activity of jogging itself. They usually run too fast to even notice the beauty of their surroundings.

Aiming for better times isn't bad, but try sometimes to run the slow way, focusing on pleasure and quality. Running is a sport for life; if your goal is to break records, you have many years ahead of you in which to get faster. But first you need to allow your body to get used to effort, to teach it basic techniques, and learn to understand your body.

We believe there is no method more enjoyable and accessible than slow jogging for living a happy and healthy life. We can't wait to see the streets and parks crowded with slow joggers of all ages. We hope that one day we will meet you somewhere, on a jogging track or maybe even at the finish line of a marathon!

Slow Jogging: References

Chapter 1

Farrell, P. A., J. H. Wilmore, E. F. Coyle, J. E. Billing, and D. L. Costill. 1979. "Plasma lactate accumulation and distance running performance." *Medicine and Science in Sports* 11 (4): 338– 44.

Chapter 2

Bramble, D. M., and D. E. Lieberman. 2004. "Endurance running and the evolution of *Homo*." *Nature* 432 (7015): 345–52.

Hreljac, A. 1993. "Preferred and energetically optimal gait transition speeds in human locomotion." *Medicine and Science in Sports and Exercise* 25 (10): 1158–62.

Raichlen, D. A., A. D. Foster, A. Seillier, A. Giuffrida, and G. L. Gerdeman. 2013. "Exercise induced endocannabinoid signaling is modulated by intensity." *European Journal of Applied Physiology* 113 (4): 869–75.

Chapter 3

Bowerman, W. J., and W. E. Harris. 1967. *Jogging*. New York, NY: Grosset & Dunlap.

Chapter 4

Tanaka, H., and M. Shindo. 1992. "The benefits of the low intensity training." *Annals of Physiological Anthropology* 11(3):365-8. Review.

Borg, G. A. 1973. "Perceived exertion: a note on 'history' and methods." *Medicine and Science in Sports* 5(2):90-3.

Chapter 5

Schnohr, P., J. H. O'Keefe, J. L. Marott, P. Lange, and G. B. Jensen. 2015. "Dose of jogging and long-term mortality: the Copenhagen City Heart Study." *Journal of the American College of Cardiology* 10 (65):411-9. 2015.

Ratey, J. J., and J. E. Loehr. 2011. "The positive impact of physical activity on cognition during adulthood: a review of underlying mechanisms, evidence and recommendations." *Review of Neuroscience* 22 (2): 171–85.

Raichlen, D. A., A. D. Foster, A. Seillier, A. Giuffrida, and G. L. Gerdeman. 2013. "Exercise induced endocannabinoid signaling is modulated by intensity." *European Journal of Applied Physiology* 113 (4): 869–75.

Michishita, R., H. Tanaka, H. Kumahara, M. Ayabe, T. Tobina, E. Yoshimura, T. Matsuda, Y. Higaki, and A. Kiyonaga. 2014. "Effects of lifestyle modifications on improvement in the blood lipid profiles in patients with dyslipidemia." *Journal of Metabolic Syndrome* 3:150. doi: 10.4172/2167-0943.1000150.

Sawada, S. S., T. Muto, H. Tanaka, I. M. Lee, R. S. Paffenbarger Jr., M. Shindo, and S. N. Blair. 2003. "Cardiorespiratory fitness and cancer mortality in Japanese men: a prospective study." *Medicine and Science in Sports and Exercise* 35(9):1546-50.

Kiyonaga, A., K. Arakawa, H. Tanaka, and M. Shindo. 1985. "Blood pressure and hormonal responses to aerobic exercise." *Hypertension* 17(1):125-31.

Motoyama, M., Y. Sunami, F. Kinoshita, A. Kiyonaga, H. Tanaka, M. Shindo, T. Irie, H. Urata, J. Sasaka, and K. Arakawa. 1998. "Blood pressure lowering effect of low intensity aerobic training in elderly hypertensive patients." *Medicine and Science in Sports and Exercise* 30(6):818-23.

Motoyama, M., Y. Sunami, F. Kinoshita, T. Irie, J. Sasaki, K. Arakawa, A. Kiyonaga, H. Tanaka, and M. Shindo. 1995. "The effects of long term low intensity aerobic training and detraining on serum lipid and lipoprotein concentrations in elderly men and women." *European Journal of Applied Physiology and Occupational Physiology* 70(2):126-31.

Sunami, Y., M. Motoyama, F. Kinoshita, Y. Mizooka, K. Sueta, A. Matsunaga, J. Sasaki, H. Tanaka, and M. Shindo. 1999. "Effects of low intensity aerobic training on the high density lipoprotein cholesterol concentration in healthy elderly subjects." *Metabolism* 48(8):984-8.

Yoshitake, T., Y. Kiyohara, I. Kato, T. Ohmura, H. Iwamoto, K. Nakayama, S. Ohmori, K. Nomiyama, H. Kawano, K. Ueda, et al. 1995. "Incidence and risk factors of vascular dementia and

Alzheimer's disease in a defined elderly Japanese population: the Hisayama Study." *Neurology* 45(6):1161-8.

Erickson, K. I., R. S. Prakash, M. W. Voss, L. Chaddock, L. Hu, K. S. Morris, S. M. White, T. R. Wójcicki, E. McAuley, and A. F. Kramer. 2009. "Aerobic fitness is associated with hippocampal volume in elderly humans." *Hippocampus.* 19(10):1030-9.

Erickson, K. I., M. W. Voss, R. S. Prakash, C. Basak, A. Szabo, L. Chaddock, J. S. Kim, et al. 2011. "Exercise training increases size of hippocampus and improves memory." *Proceedings of the National Academy of Sciences of the United States of America* 15;108(7):3017-22.

Harada, T., S. Okagawa, and K. Kubota. 2004. "Jogging improved performance of a behavioral branching task: implications for prefrontal activation." *Neuroscience Research* 49(3):325-37.

Chapter 6

Margaria, R., P. Cerreteteli, P. Aghemo, and G. Sassi. 1963. "Energy cost of running." *Journal of Applied Physiology* 18:367-70.

Mayer, J., and D. W. Thomas. 1967. "Regulation of food intake and obesity." *Science* 21;156(3773):328-37. Review.

Mayer, J., N. B. Marshal, J. J. Vitale, J. H. Christensen, M. B. Mashayekhi, and F. J. Stare. 1954. "Exercise, food intake and body weight in normal rats and genetically obese adult mice." *American Journal of Physiology* 177(3):544-8.

Michishita, R., H. Tanaka, H. Kumahara, M. Ayabe, T. Tobina, E. Yoshimura, T. Matsuda, Y. Higaki, and Kiyonaga. 2014. "Effects of lifestyle modifications on improvement in the blood lipid profiles in patients with dyslipidemia." *Journal of Metabolic Syndrome* 3:150. doi: 10.4172/2167-0943.1000150.

Yoshimura, E., H. Kumahara, T. Tobina, T. Matsuda, M. Ayabe, A. Kiyonaga, K. Anzai, Y. Higaki, and H. Tanaka. 2014 "Lifestyle intervention involving calorie restriction with or without aerobic exercise training improves liver fat in adults with visceral adiposity." *Journal of Obesity.* 197216. doi: 10.1155/2014/197216. Epub 2014. Apr 17.

Chapter 7

Mori, Y., M. Ayabe, T. Yahiro, T. Tobina, A. Kiyonaga, and M. Shindo. 2006. "The effect of home-based bench step exercise on aerobic capacity, lower extremity power and static balance in older adults." *International Journal of Sport and Health Science* 4:1–7 10.

Chapter 8

Murakami, I., T. Sakuragi, H. Uemura, H. Menda, M. Shindo, and H. Tanaka. 2012. "Significant effect of a pre-exercise high fat meal after a 3 day high carbohydrate diet on endurance performance." *Nutrients* Jul;4(7):625-37.

Tanaka, H., J. Cléroux, J. de Champlain, J. R. Ducharme, and R. Collu. 1986. "Persistent effects of a marathon run on the pituitary testicular axis." *Journal of Endocrinological Investigation* 9(2):97-101.

Chapter 9

Tobina, T., K. Yoshioka, A. Hirata, S. Mori, A. Kiyonaga, and H. Tanaka. 2011. "Peroxisomal proliferator activated receptor gamma co-activator alpha gene expression increases above the lactate threshold in human skeletal muscle." *Journal of Sports Medicine and Physical Fitness* 51(4):683-8.

Nishida, Y., H. Tanaka, T. Tobina, K. Murakami, N. Shono, M. Shindo, W. Ogawa, M. Yoshioka, and J. St. Amand. 2010. "Regulation of muscle genes by moderate exercise." *International Journal of Sports Medicine* Sept:31(9):656-70.

Puigserver, P., Z. Wu, C. W. Park, R. Graves, M. Wright, and B. M. Spiegelman. 1998. "A cold inducible coactivator of nuclear receptors linked to adaptive thermogenesis." *Cell* 20;92(6):829-39.

Tabata, I., K. Nishimura, M. Kouzaki, Y. Hirai, F. Ogita, M. Miyachi, and K. Yamamoto. 1996. "Effects of moderate intensity endurance and high intensity intermittent training on anaerobic capacity and VO2max." *Medicine and Science in Sports and Exercise* 28(10):1327-30.

Terada, S., K. Kawanaka, M. Goto, T. Shimokawa, and I. Tabata. 2005. "Effects of high intensity intermittent swimming on PGC 1alpha protein expression in rat skeletal muscle." *Acta Physiologica Scandinavica* 184(1):59-65.

Gibala, M. J., and S. L. McGee. 2008. "Metabolic adaptations to short-term high-intensity interval training: a little pain for a lot of gain?" *Exercise and Sport Sciences Reviews* 36(2): 58–63.

Hansen, A. K., C. P. Fisher, P. Plomgaard, J. L. Andersen, B. Saltin, and B. K. Pedersen. 2005. "Skeletal muscle adaptation: training twice every second day vs. training once daily." *Journal of Applied Physiology* 98: 93–99.

Yeo, W. K., C. D. Paton, A. P. Garnham, L. M. Burke, A. L. Carey, and J. A. Hawley. 2008. "Skeletal muscle adaptation and performance responses to once a day versus twice every second day endurance training regimens." *Journal of Applied Physiology* 105(5):1462-70.

Almond, C. S., A. Y. Shin, E. B. Fortescue, R. C. Mannix, D. Wypij, B. A. Binstadt, C. N. Duncan, D. P. Olson, A. E. Salerno, J. W. Newburger, and D. S. Greenes. 2005. "Hyponatremia among runners in the Boston Marathon." *New England Journal of Medicine* 352(15):1550-6.

For More Information About the Slow Jogging Movement

To help you make the most of your slow jogging experience and support you in reaching your goals, we have created various goods—from shoes designed especially for slow jogging, to sets of songs that will provide perfect pacing and relaxing sounds on your everyday jog. You can sample and get them on Amazon at "Slow Jogging Della."

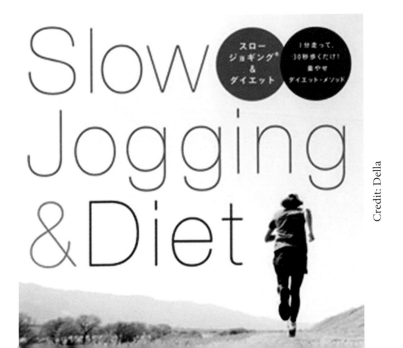

Credit: Della

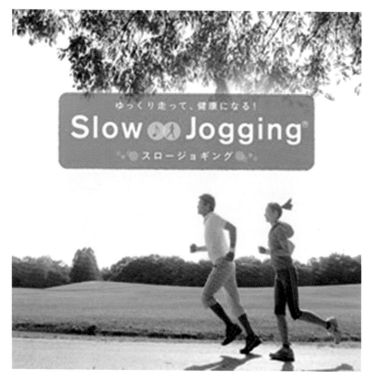

Credit: Della

You can also look for "Slow Jogging" in the iTunes store.

We also organize slow jogging events, workshops, training camps, and diet retreats in Japan and worldwide.

To ask questions and get all the newest information on the slow jogging movement, visit us at www.facebook.com/slowjogginginternational/ or contact us directly at jackowska.magda@gmail.com.

We are looking forward to hearing from you!

Acknowledgments

We would like to thank Professors Emeritus Munehiro Shindo and Shigeru Obara and all the current and past colleagues and students of Fukuoka University Institute for Physical Activity for years of joint efforts in slow jogging studies and promotion.

We would like to thank our families for their continued support and encouragement.

Last but not least, we thank Dr. Mark Cucuzzella and Bill Katovsky of the Natural Running Center—without you this book wouldn't have found its way to the United States!